THE BODY PLAN PLUS EXERCISE PROGRAMME

We all come in different shapes & sizes and have various levels of stamina, fitness and flexibility.
Which is why....The Body Plan Plus Exercise programme has been created to cater for all body types.

This Exercise Plan is really clever and has been designed to allow you to jump in and get started at any level. You pick the starting point and exercises that are right for you!

Increase your fitness levels at the pace your body will thank you for. Burn those calories every day without burning yourself out and quitting!

I do not know you personally, and do not know your current weight, levels of fitness or flexibility.
So if you feel like I have under-estimated your ability in any way I apologise.

The Body Plan Plus Exercise Programme is more of a formula than a routine. I am not going to tell you which exercises to do, that's up to you with your honest approach.

I do have a suggested starting point for your body type, and again if you feel my suggested starting point is not enough for you, then please accept my apology.

The next few pages explain my exercise formula for progressive increases. The first time you read through, it may look complicated, but trust me it isn't. Read it through a couple of times and watch the video linked to our Facebook page or website: www.the**body**plan**plus**.com

This formula is easy, and your body will be grateful you're using it!

The exercises are shown on the next few pages. Molly the model comes in three body types, A, B and C. For illustration purposes, I am using Molly the model Body Type A.

"We are as trees. To be found in all shapes and sizes.
Although different, we are all beautiful"

WHY DOES THIS PROGRAMME WORK SO WELL?

To put it in a nut shell, it's a clever progressive routine that works with your body. Soon you will agree that it's the best exercise programme around. When using this system your body will tell you when to move on to the next level. When your body is doing the talking, you're doing it right.

You can't over do it with this programme, you should only move on to the next level when you have ticked "Completed" five times in a row.

Your body will slowly get used to the increases of resistance. In a short time you will increase your stamina, fitness levels and lose weight dramatically without feeling tired or fatigued. Feeling fatigued the day after exercising is what makes people give up! This should not happen with The Body Plan Plus Exercise Programme!

OK! SO HOW DOES IT ALL WORK?

The Body Plan Plus Exercise Routine For Progressive Resistance over time.

When you are ready to make your workouts harder, you will be:

- **STEP 1**   Adding Exercises
- **STEP 2**   Adding Sets
- **STEP 3**   Increasing Exercise Time
- **STEP 4**   Reducing Resting Time
- **STEP 5**   Adding Higher Level Exercises

You only make your workouts harder when you have completed five cycles of your current routine. You must have a tick in every **SET** box five times in a row. This is fully explained over the next few pages.

Exercising makes you thirsty and hungry. Drink plenty of water during your workout and always have a post workout snack… something filling, healthy and low in calories. This will take away the hunger feeling that you would normally get a few hours after putting your body through stress.

YOUR STARTING POINT

Your suggested starting point is

- 2 Exercises (Chosen for your recommended body type)
- 3 Sets of each Exercise
- 45 Seconds for your Exercise Time
- 60 Seconds for your Resting Time

* You may think this is not enough exercise time for you? You may be right, you may be wrong. Let's see how you feel when you have completed the first session. If you feel it isn't enough, simply add another SET on your next workout day until you get the balance right for you.

Choose your exercises with a Star Level Difficultly Rating of 1 or 2 (**See list of exercises**)

Other than Stair Walking and Free Squats, you should perform your exercises as quick as possible, providing it is safe to do so. "**Don't go crazy, just a nice steady pace**"

| Exercise Time | |
Perform your exercise within your **Exercise Time Goal** "No More, No Less"

| Resting Time | |
Rest only for your **Resting Time Goal** "No More, No Less"

   * *Don't worry if you can't match your exercise time just yet - See Step backwards Page*

You should be able to keep track of your times, using your smart phone or a stopwatch.

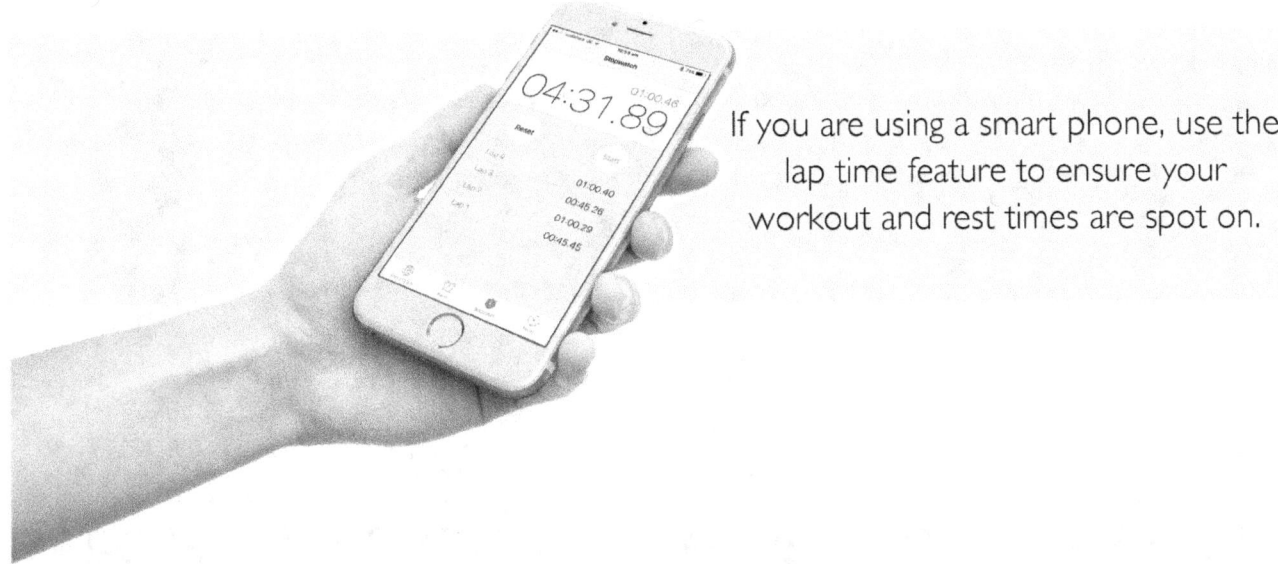

If you are using a smart phone, use the lap time feature to ensure your workout and rest times are spot on.

YOUR EXERCISE LOG OVERVIEW

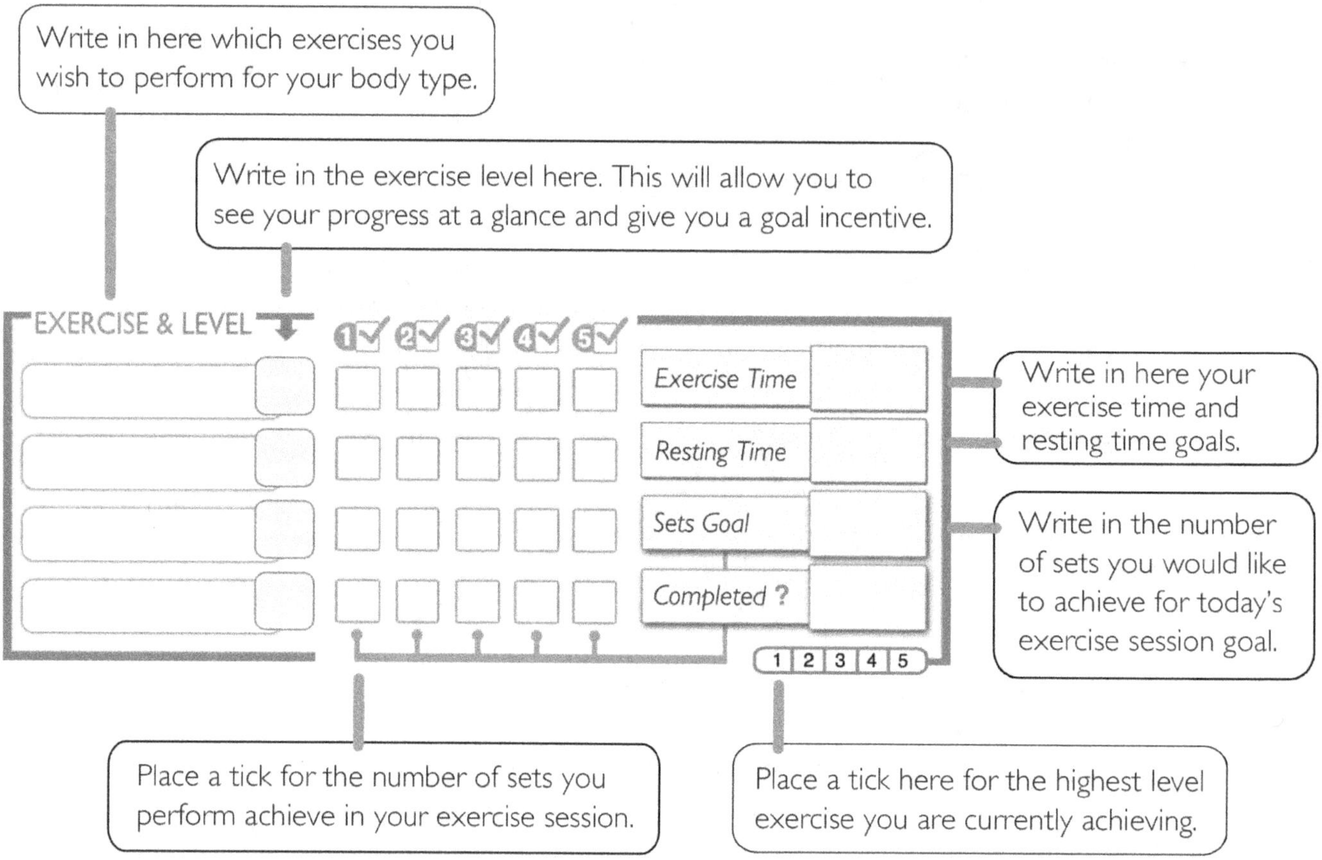

Write in here which exercises you wish to perform for your body type.

Write in the exercise level here. This will allow you to see your progress at a glance and give you a goal incentive.

EXERCISE & LEVEL

1 ✓ 2 ✓ 3 ✓ 4 ✓ 5 ✓

Exercise Time

Resting Time

Sets Goal

Completed ?

1 | 2 | 3 | 4 | 5

Write in here your exercise time and resting time goals.

Write in the number of sets you would like to achieve for today's exercise session goal.

Place a tick for the number of sets you perform achieve in your exercise session.

Place a tick here for the highest level exercise you are currently achieving.

The Body Plan Plus exercise system is a unique formula that allows you to progress slowly over time and listening to your body. On the next few pages I will show you how to increase your intensity over time.

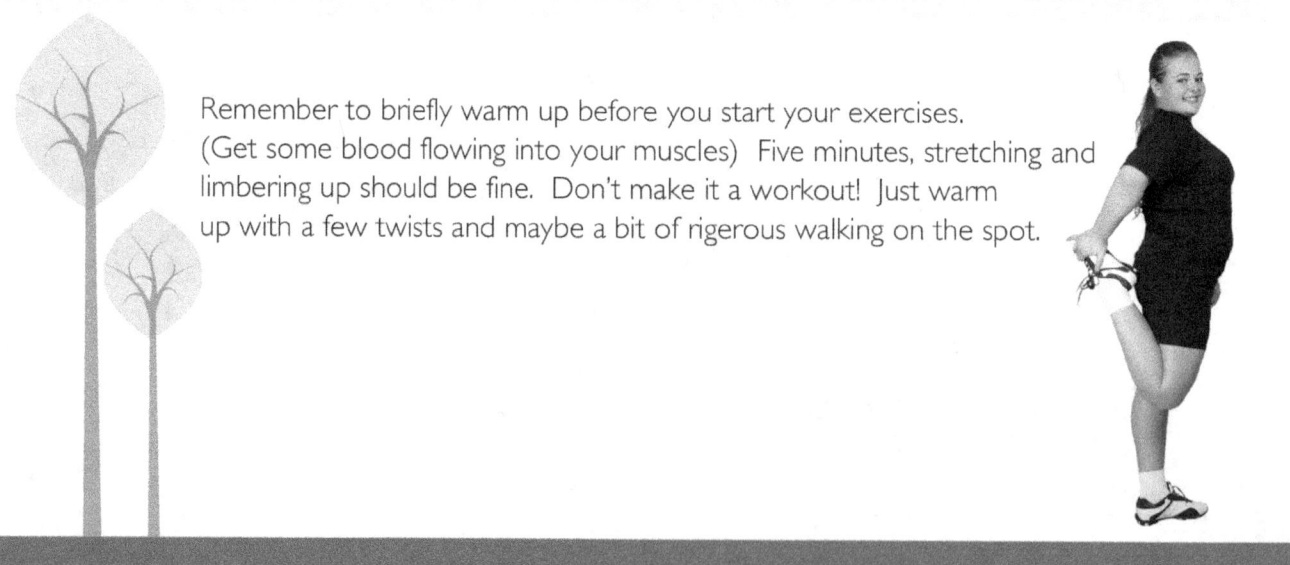

Remember to briefly warm up before you start your exercises. (Get some blood flowing into your muscles) Five minutes, stretching and limbering up should be fine. Don't make it a workout! Just warm up with a few twists and maybe a bit of rigerous walking on the spot.

STEP 1 ADDING EXERCISES

YOUR TRAINING LOG WILL LOOK LIKE THIS WHEN YOU START (2 EXERCISES)

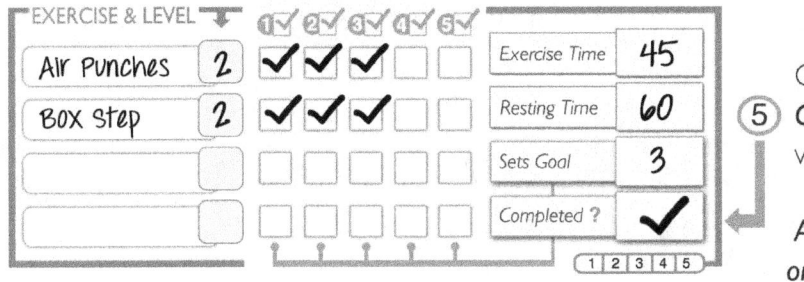

Continue with this routine until you have **(5) Completed** five ticks over a five day workout period.

After a week you should be ready to move on and add an extra exercise to your routine.

YOUR TRAINING LOG WILL LOOK LIKE THIS AFTER WEEK 1 (3 EXERCISES)

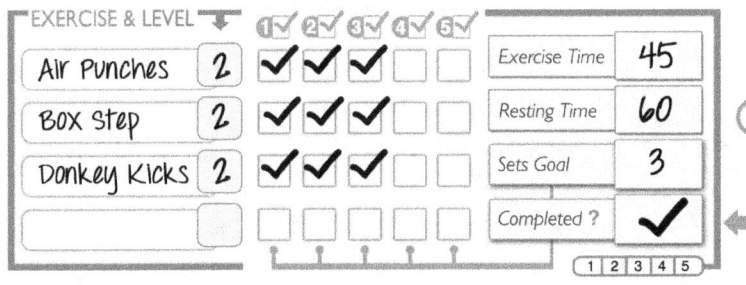

Continue with this routine until you have **(5) Completed** five ticks over a five day workout period.

After a week you should be ready to move on and add an extra exercise to your routine.

YOUR TRAINING LOG WILL LOOK LIKE THIS AFTER WEEK 2 (4 EXERCISES)

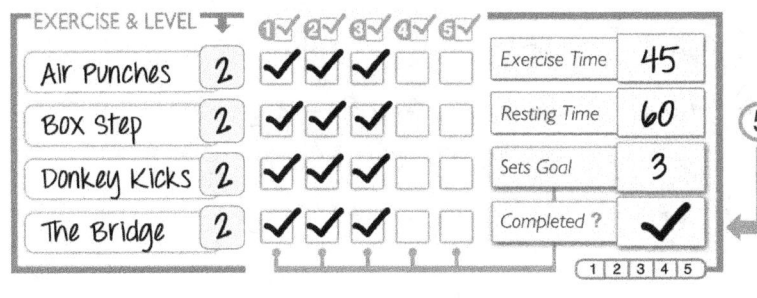

Continue with this routine until you have **(5) Completed** five ticks over a five day workout period.

After a week you should be ready to move on and add an extra exercise to your routine.

STEP 2 ADDING SETS

Well done! You're performing 4 Exercises Per Workout! It's time to add some sets.

When you have completed your five ticks in a row for performing 4 exercises it's time
for **STEP 2** (Adding Sets) Add 1 Set for each Exercise, and follow the same rule. Do not add
another set until you have completed 5 consecutive ticks in your "Completed Box".

Follow this cycle until you are performing 5 Sets for each exercise.

It may have taken you up to 3 to 4 Weeks to get this far, but by now your body is becoming used
 to the extra effort and you will begin to feel the changes.

- Your body is becoming more toned and muscles stronger
- Your Heart is becoming stronger and pumping blood faster
- You are burning more calories and losing more body fat at a faster pace

When adding sets your Log Sheets will look like this:

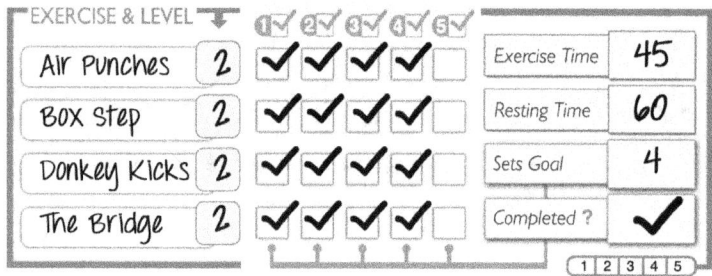

FOUR EXERCISES (4 SETS)

Exercise time goal (45 Seconds)
Resting time goal (60 Seconds)

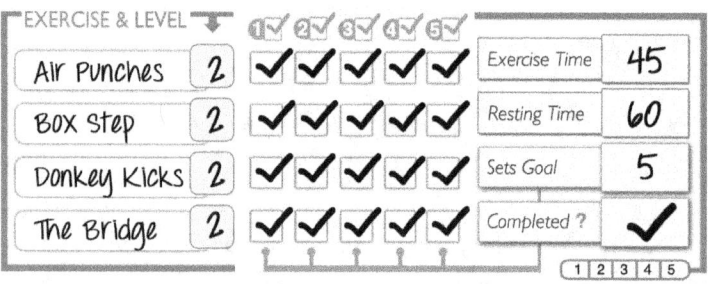

FOUR EXERCISES (5 SETS)

Exercise time goal (45 Seconds)
Resting time goal (60 Seconds)

STEP 3 INCREASING YOUR EXERCISE TIME

Now you are performing 5 Sets for each of your exercises. It's time to move onto **STEP 3**

Your exercise time has always been set to 45 Seconds. It's now time to increase this time to 60 Seconds.

This is an extra 15 Seconds Per Exercise. In total this works out to be an additional 5 minutes exercise time for your routine.

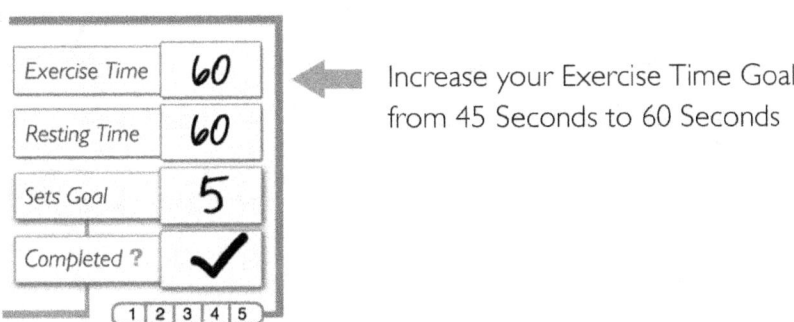

Increase your Exercise Time Goal from 45 Seconds to 60 Seconds

Remember the Golden Rule! Do not increase to the next step until you have completed 5 Ticks in a row.

STEP 4 REDUCING YOUR RESTING TIME

Your resting time has always been set to 60 Seconds. It's now time to reduce this time to 45 Seconds. This is a reduction of 15 Seconds Per Exercise. In total this reduces your resting time a further 5 minutes.

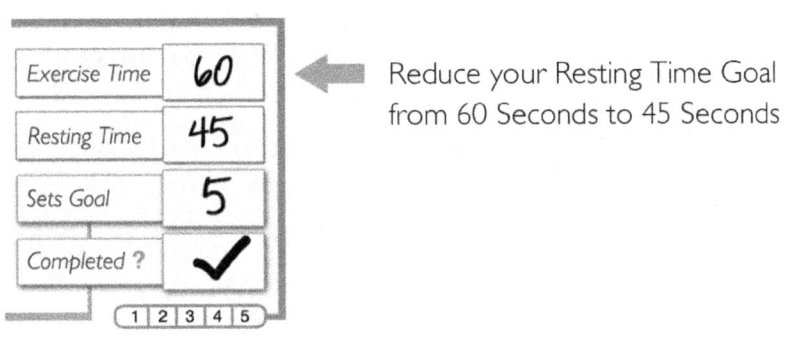

Reduce your Resting Time Goal from 60 Seconds to 45 Seconds

STEP 5 HIGHER LEVEL EXERCISES

You have worked your way up and are now performing:

- 4 Exercises
- 5 Sets of Each Exercise
- 60 Seconds Exercise Time
- 45 Seconds Resting Time

It is time to choose some higher level exercises from your list.   Choose one that is of a higher level of intensity and difficulty.   Once again, following the Golden Rule, don't add a higher level exercise until you have completed 5 Ticks in a row from your previous **STEP**…

The highest Level you can reach with The Body Plan Exercise Programme will look like this:

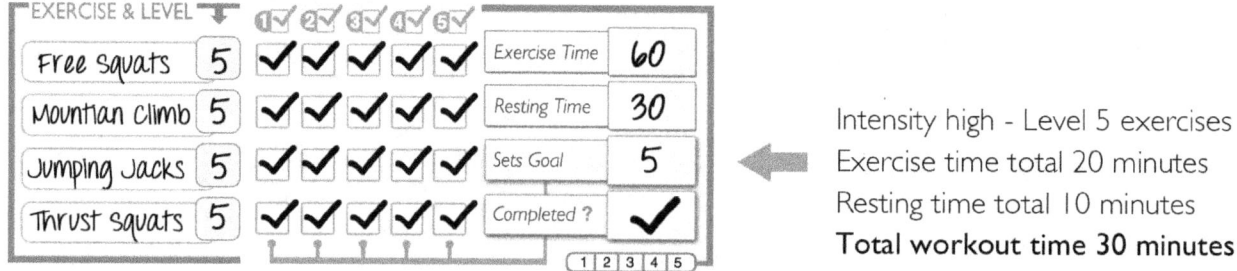

Intensity high - Level 5 exercises
Exercise time total 20 minutes
Resting time total 10 minutes
Total workout time 30 minutes

      AND if you can do this, you are **SUPER FIT**….!

When you get familiar with this Programmes structure, you can play around with all the STEPS and really mix things up a bit. You can alter your Exercise and Resting Time Goals, change your exercises to something different for every workout.   Or you can perform lower amounts of sets for higher level Exercise.   You choose and make your Exercise Plan completely personal for you.

Take a break….
If you want to continue getting fitter and losing more body fat, simply stick with it.
But, **NEVER** do more than your body can cope with. When you have built up to performing five sets - Take a day off - Maybe Wednesdays.

If you feel tired and achy on the mornings after your workout, use the system but in reverse. - **STEP BACKWARDS** and follow the cycle again until you stop feeling fatigued the following day.

STEP FORWARD OR TAKE A STEP BACKWARDS

The goal for this Programme, is for you to just keep doing more, without feeling the pain of it all. The aim of the Body Plan Plus Programme is to increase your physical activity and intensity gently over time, and therefore get you fitter, stronger, healthier and losing even more weight.

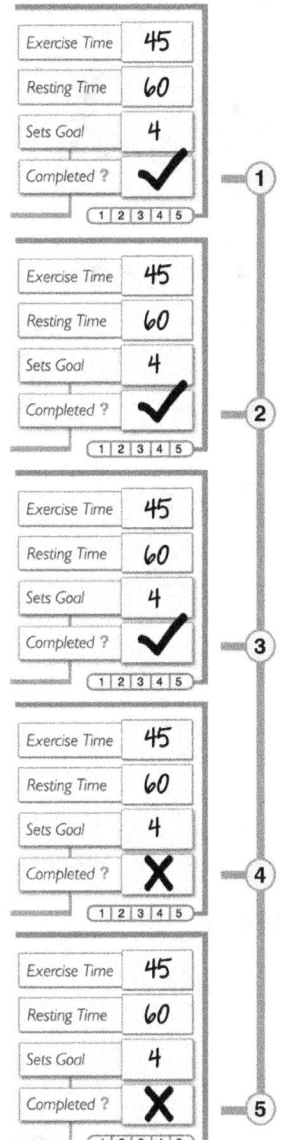

Even this programme can feel like it's too much sometimes if you push yourself too hard. So you need to know when to move forward and if needed **move backwards** a step. This is how to work it out to ensure your listening to your body.

When you have completed your entire routine, hitting your Exercise Time Goal and Resting Time Goal, place a tick in the box.

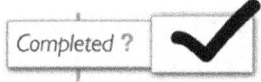

WHEN TO PUT AN "X"

- If you fail to complete all your sets
- If you have to rest longer then your Resting Time Goal
- If you Exercise for less then your Exercise Time Goal

When you don't manage to complete your entire routine for any of these reasons. Follow the same routine the following week. (*After a weekend break you may be able to nail it next time.*)

If you don't manage to complete your routine again the following week "STEP BACK"

To step back do the following:

Change your Exercise to a less intense one **Or......** Keep the same Exercises, but reduce the Exercise Time by 15 Seconds and increase your resting time by 15 Seconds.

Then continue on for the next week. And if you then hit your "3 ticks in a row" Go back to the same Exercises and Goal Times as before. You will soon get the hang of it and be slowly adapting your body to these changes. You will be surprised when you look back over the weeks to see how much you have advanced and how much fitter you feel.

WINDMILLS

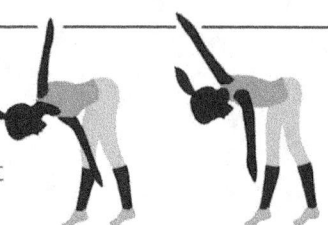

Bend forward with your arms straight and twist your body and point to your toes. Your right arm pointing to your left toe, and left arm to your right. Swing your body quite quickly. You don't have to touch your toes, simply point to them. Over time if you repeat this exercise, try getting closer to your toes.

DANCE CRAZY

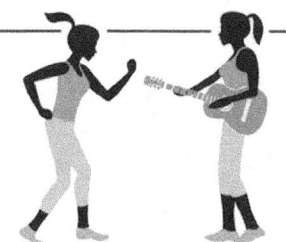

Imagine you are your favourite pop idol and on stage. Go mental and dance around with all the energy you have. Produce a performance that the crowd will appreciate. Play your guitar, bash your drums and dance crazy.

SOFA SQUATS

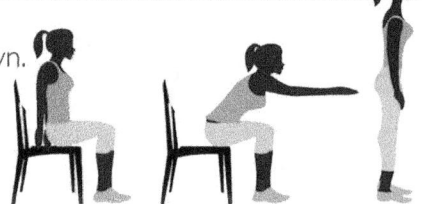

As it says "on the tin" From a seated position, stand up and then sit down. Perform as fast as possible and swing your arms out to aid in your stand up motion. You can remain seated for 1 to 2 seconds if required.

THE PLANK

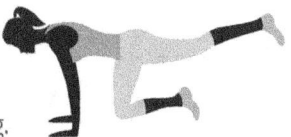

Get into the pushup position on the floor. How bend your elbows and rest your weight on your forearms. Your elbows should be directly beneath your shoulders, and keeping your body in a straight line without raising your bum. Hold this position for your specified time.

KICK BACKS

Start on all-fours. Your knees should be slightly hip width apart, as shown. Using one leg, raise it straight above your bottom with a slight bend in the knee, then bring it back to the starting point position. Repeat with the other leg.

HALF JACKS

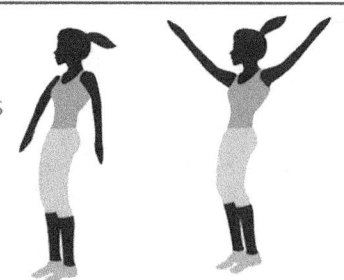

jumping jacks get your heart pumping. Bend your knees to get the spring, but instead of jumping with your feet wide apart, only jump with them a few inches apart. In time when you get used to the movement you can jump with your feet wider apart. Continue this patten over time until you are performing a standard jumping jack.

QUARTER SQUATS

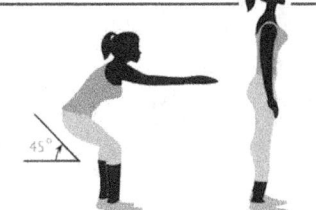

The same as a squat, but instead of lowering yourself so your thighs are parallel to the floor, you only squat to about 45 degrees. You will feel the tension in your thighs and this is what counts. As you get used to this movement you can extend your range until you are performing a full squat.

STAIR WALKING

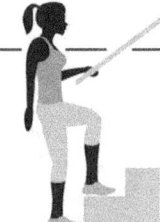

As it says "on the tin" Try and move at a faster pace than normal. Keep your hand on the hand rail and let the rail run through your hands to keep you safe and steady.

AIR PUNCHES

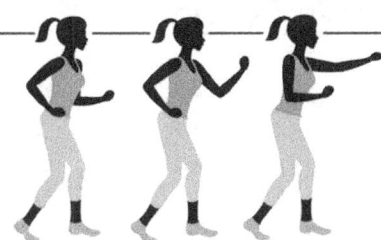

Imagine you're in a Boxing ring and you're punching your opponent in the head and body. Move around as if in the ring and avoid their counter punches by bobbing, ducking and weaving around. Throw your punches as quick as you can..

HIGH KNEES

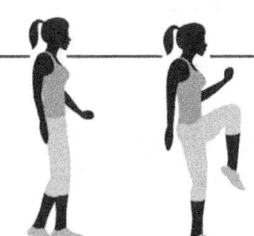

Just like jogging on the spot, but raise your knees as high as you can. Perform this exercise as fast as you can without losing your balance. Support yourself with a chair if required.

THE BRIDGE

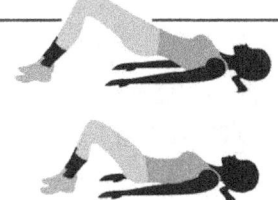

As shown, lay flat on the floor with your feet about 12inches apart from your bottom. Raise your hips into the air to form a bridge with your body. Hold this position for a second or two. Lower and repeat.

BOX STEPS

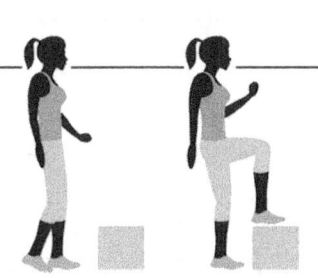

From a standing position take one step on and one step off. Use the bottom step of your stairs. Repeat as fast as possible without losing your balance.

LUNGES

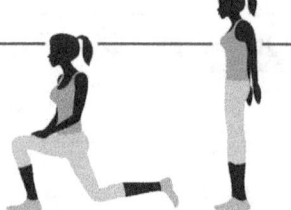

From a standing position, lunge forward on one leg until your thigh is parallel with the floor. Place your hands on your thigh for balance. Thrust yourself back into the starting position and repeat.

FREE SQUATS

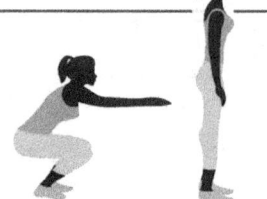

From a standing position, squat down until your thighs are parallel with floor. You can hold this position for a second or two before returning to the starting position.

KNEE/PUSH UPS

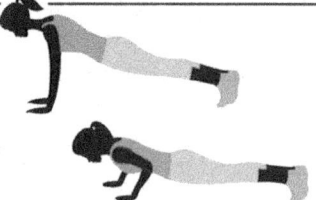

Perform a standard push up or knee push up.
The same as regular push ups, but your body weight is on your knees instead of your toes. Lower yourself down until your chest touches the floor and push yourself back up into the starting position.

LEG RAISES

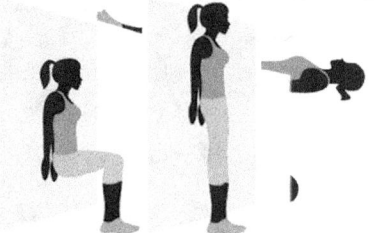

In a lying position, raise your legs about 12 inches from the floor, hold for seconds and repeat. Use your arms for balance and to aid the movement A small beanbag will aid you. If you feel pain in your middle or lower back stop this exercise until your flexibility and strength has improved.

WALL SQUATS

From a standing position, lean against the wall and squat down until your thighs are parallel with the floor. You can hold this position for a second or two before returning to the starting position. This movement is harder than you think, and you may find free squats easier to perform.

CRUNCHES

From a lying position raise your head and legs at the same time, as shown. This is a very difficult and taxing exercise to perform correctly. You can cheat a little and already have your feet raised on a bean bag, large cushion or edge of your sofa.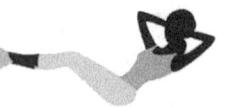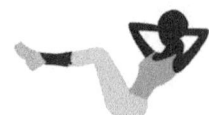

JUMPING JACKS

From a standing upright position, jump into a star position with your legs parallel with your shoulders. Clap your hands above your head and then instantly jump back to the starting position.

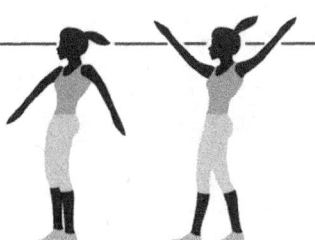

THRUST SQUATS

From a standing position, squat down and place your hands on the floor between your knees and thrust your legs back into the plank position. In one continuous movement thrust your legs back into the squat position and then jump up and repeat.

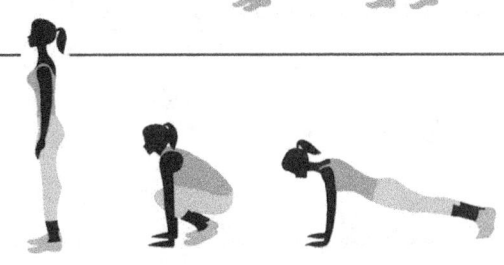

MOUNTAIN CLIMBS

From the starting PLANK position, thrust your legs alternatively up to your chest in a running motion or "climbing motion"

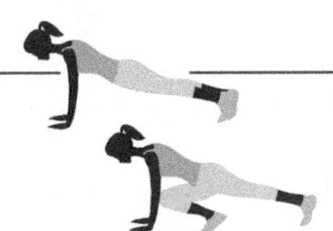

CREATE YOUR OWN EXERCISES

Exercise is about movement and making your muscles work a little harder than normal. Muscles respond and burn energy from repetition (Continuous movement) and or tension from lifting weight (Force against gravity) Your body is weight, so therefore various movements force your body to act against gravity.

For example: Getting up from a sitting position causes your thigh muscles to contract as you put your upper body weight on them! Your thigh muscles have to contract for just a moment, but if you repeat the process continuously they will call upon more energy to keep the movement going - The heavier you are, the greater the force against gravity and the harder your thigh muscles will have to work, and thus burn more energy.

A lighter person could perform more repetitions than a heaver person. So once again, not all exercises are equal, and it looks like the larger person just isn't putting in the effort - But believe me they are, if not more!

If you are heavier or have limited flexibility, you can take an existing exercise movement, and reduce its range of motion to make it easier and fair. Remember, it's all relative and the effort required matches your body weight and structure, so the calorie burning is equal to the amount of energy you require to work against gravity.

I have invented two new exercises that do this. People with lower flexibly or heavier bodies will be able perform these moves more comfortably and burn just as many calories, if not more! **Half Jacks** (An easier version of jumping jacks) and **Quarter Squats** (An easier version of squating) See Body Plan exercises page 186

Feel free to create and invent your own exercises. All you have to do is ensure your muscles are under tension, and tire if you repeat the movement many times. If you invent an exercise that you can do pretty fast, without losing balance - then that's even better! Let me know the mechanics of your new exercise and I will put them up on our Facebook for others to try.

Remember, exercise is not about working out to complete exhaustion! Getting fit, increasing your stamina and all round health will come fasterwith repetition. Exercising lightly, every day or as many days possible willbe more beneficial than a burst of "Over doing it".

Pushing yourself beyond your limits is a common mistake and will simply produce - negative results! No matter how fit you are!

Don't Panic!
"I Feel Fine"

SUMMARY WHERE DO YOU GO FROM HERE?

Weight loss and fitness is a continuous endeavour. In the beginning it can seem like a real challenge and your will power may be tested on many occasions. It is a bit like everything in life and when you are the beginning it's hard and maybe a little scary! Over time you become the master of it and it becomes easy and fun. It really does!

It's a wonderful "Catch 22", the fitter and thinner you become the more you want to push yourself. The more you push yourself the healthier you get!

It really will happen for you to! Remember, small honest steps first. Know your body and what it's capable of. Listen to your body and don't change too much to soon, because if you do you could potentially fail.

In time you will want to do more exercise and take the longer routes. Calorie burning tasks from house work to gardening will no longer seem a challenge. In fact you will not notice walking mile after mile and everything becomes easy to achieve.

I haven't even mentioned the new wardrobe yet! - I will leave this for you to experience!

Keep it up, keep tracking your foods and recording your exercise progress. Think of yourself as a growing tree - throughout the difficulties that lay in your path, you will flourish and

YOU ARE BEAUTIFUL!

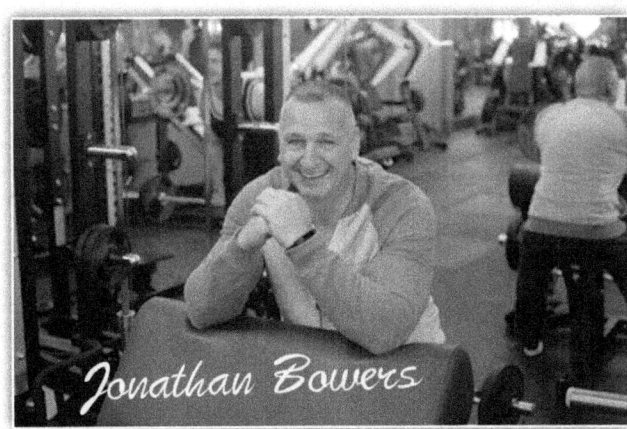

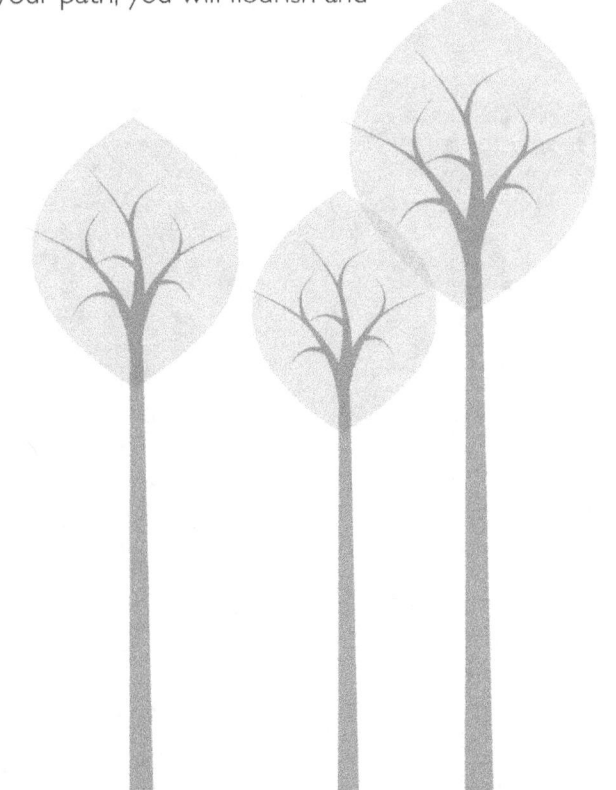

Any questions or queries, please don't hesitate to get in contact.

If you like this exercise training dairy, then you will love
The Body Plan Plus,
Food Diary, Planner & Exercise plan for everyone!

www.thebodyplanplus.com

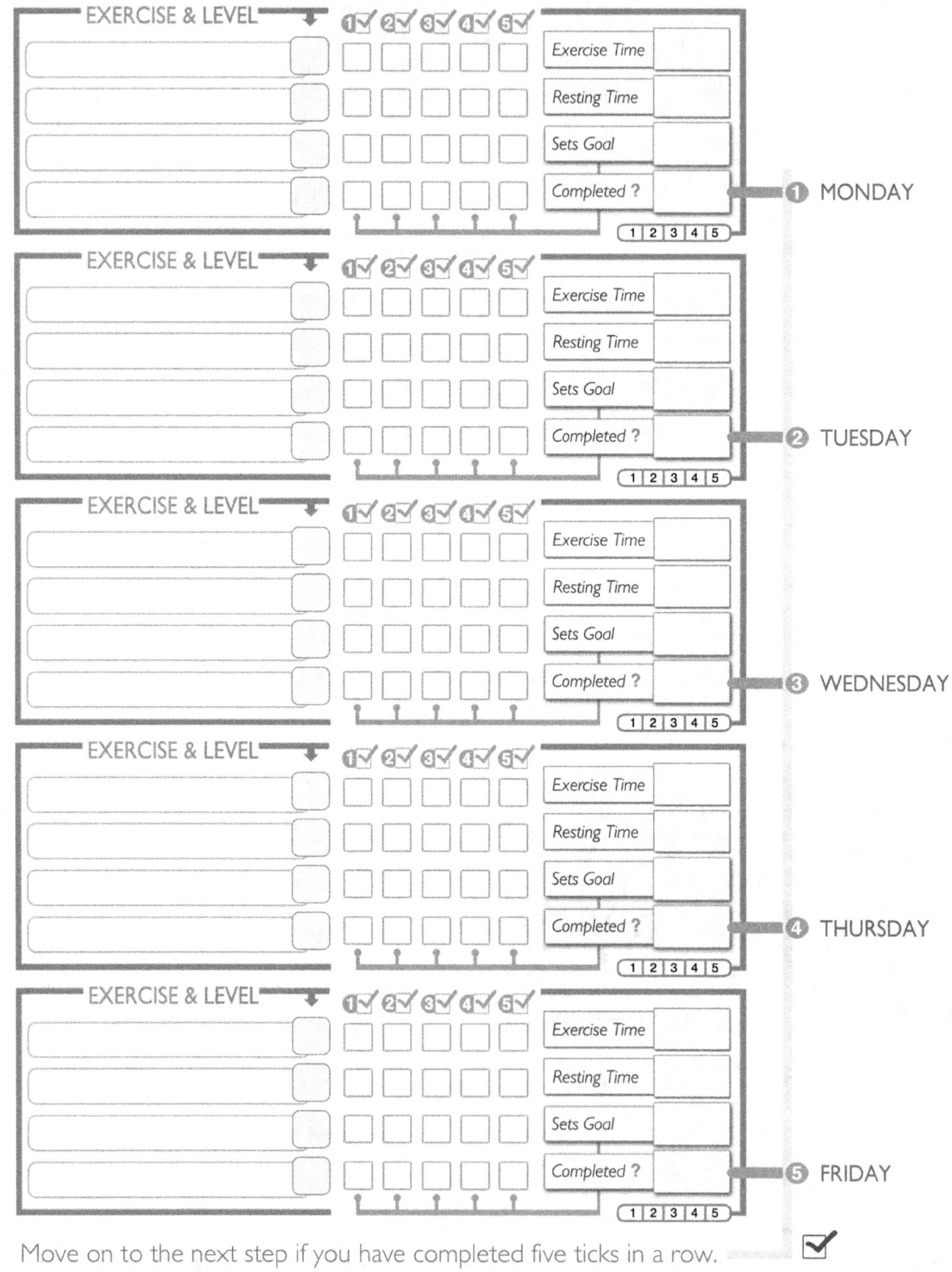

EXERCISE & LEVEL

1 ✓ 2 ✓ 3 ✓ 4 ✓ 5 ✓

Exercise Time

Resting Time

Sets Goal

Completed ?

1 2 3 4 5

① MONDAY

② TUESDAY

③ WEDNESDAY

④ THURSDAY

⑤ FRIDAY

Move on to the next step if you have completed five ticks in a row. ☑

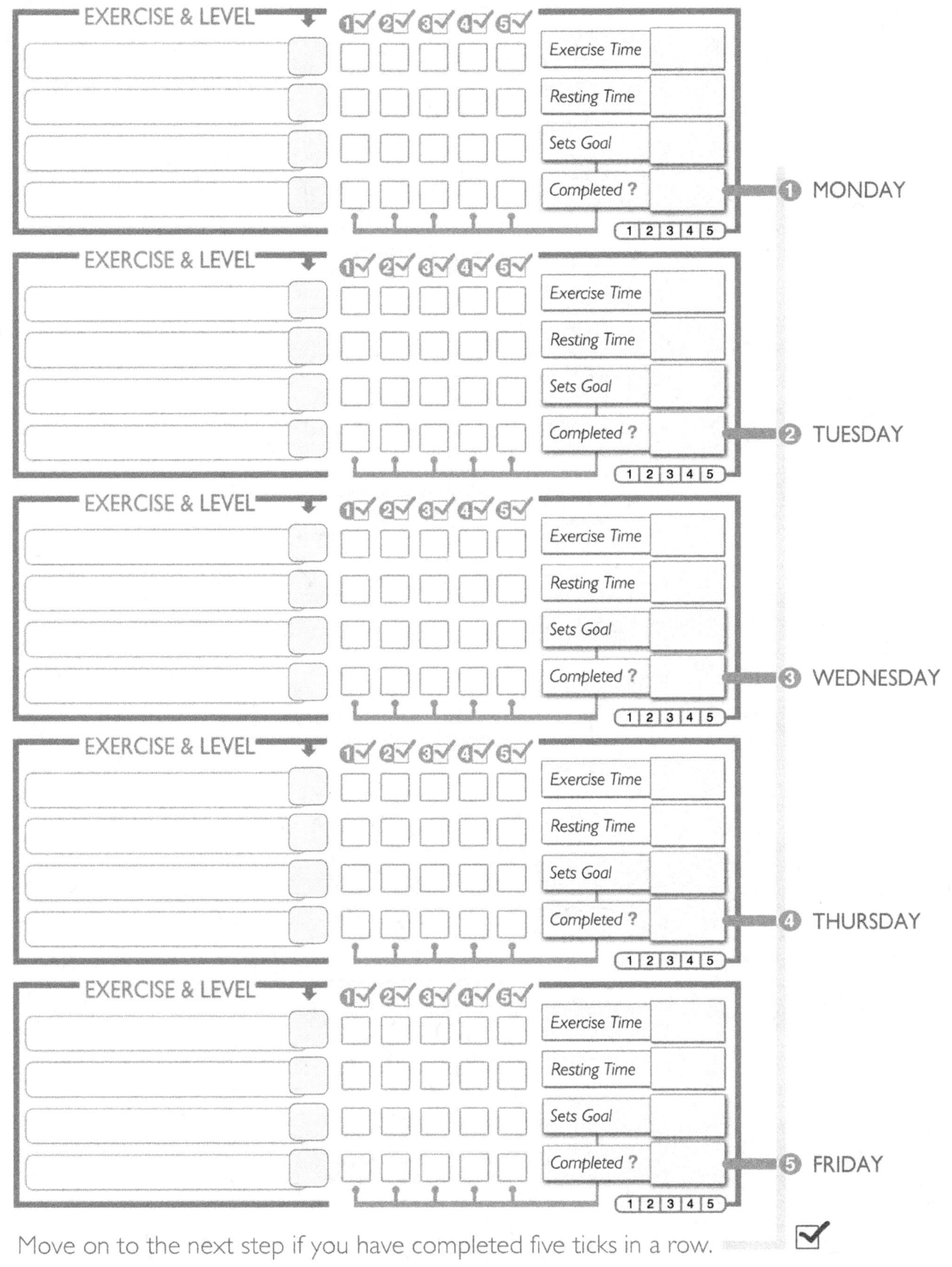

EXERCISE & LEVEL   ❶✓ ❷✓ ❸✓ ❹✓ ❺✓

Exercise Time
Resting Time
Sets Goal
Completed ?

1 2 3 4 5

❶ MONDAY

EXERCISE & LEVEL   ❶✓ ❷✓ ❸✓ ❹✓ ❺✓

Exercise Time
Resting Time
Sets Goal
Completed ?

1 2 3 4 5

❷ TUESDAY

EXERCISE & LEVEL   ❶✓ ❷✓ ❸✓ ❹✓ ❺✓

Exercise Time
Resting Time
Sets Goal
Completed ?

1 2 3 4 5

❸ WEDNESDAY

EXERCISE & LEVEL   ❶✓ ❷✓ ❸✓ ❹✓ ❺✓

Exercise Time
Resting Time
Sets Goal
Completed ?

1 2 3 4 5

❹ THURSDAY

EXERCISE & LEVEL   ❶✓ ❷✓ ❸✓ ❹✓ ❺✓

Exercise Time
Resting Time
Sets Goal
Completed ?

1 2 3 4 5

❺ FRIDAY

Move on to the next step if you have completed five ticks in a row. ✓

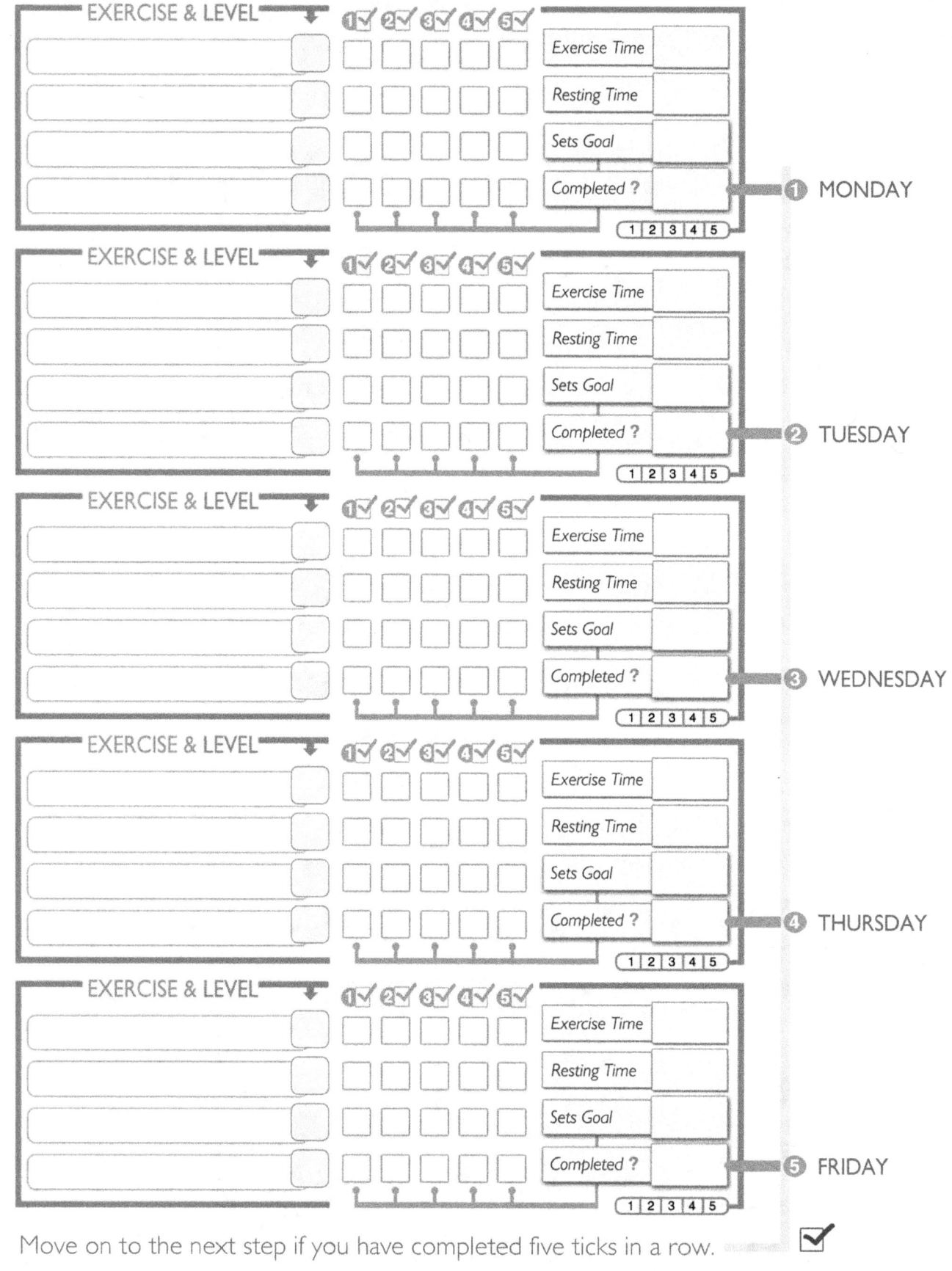

EXERCISE & LEVEL

1☑ 2☑ 3☑ 4☑ 5☑

Exercise Time

Resting Time

Sets Goal

Completed ?

1 2 3 4 5

❶ MONDAY

EXERCISE & LEVEL

1☑ 2☑ 3☑ 4☑ 5☑

Exercise Time

Resting Time

Sets Goal

Completed ?

1 2 3 4 5

❷ TUESDAY

EXERCISE & LEVEL

1☑ 2☑ 3☑ 4☑ 5☑

Exercise Time

Resting Time

Sets Goal

Completed ?

1 2 3 4 5

❸ WEDNESDAY

EXERCISE & LEVEL

1☑ 2☑ 3☑ 4☑ 5☑

Exercise Time

Resting Time

Sets Goal

Completed ?

1 2 3 4 5

❹ THURSDAY

EXERCISE & LEVEL

1☑ 2☑ 3☑ 4☑ 5☑

Exercise Time

Resting Time

Sets Goal

Completed ?

1 2 3 4 5

❺ FRIDAY

Move on to the next step if you have completed five ticks in a row. ☑

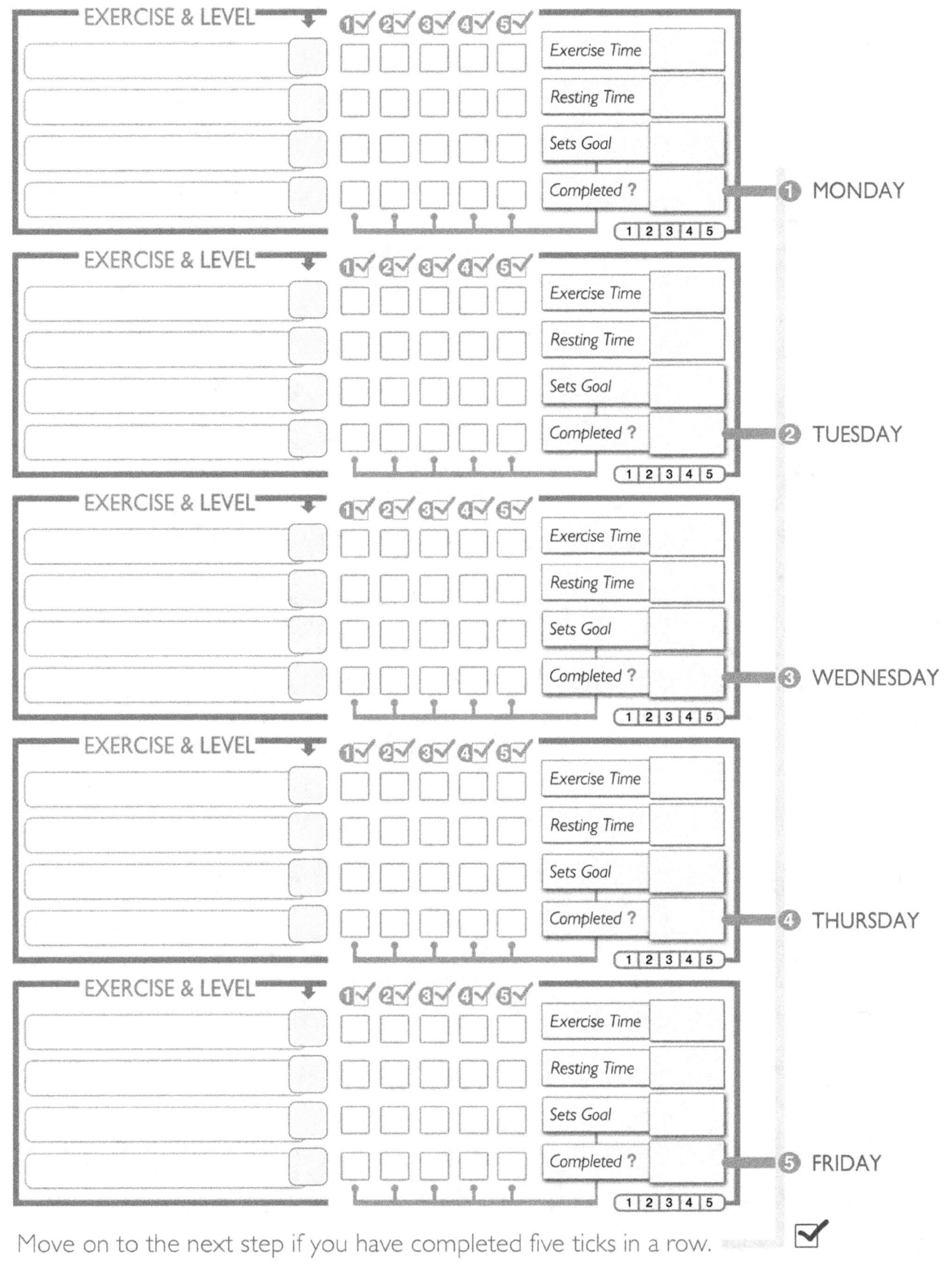

EXERCISE & LEVEL

① ② ③ ④ ⑤

Exercise Time

Resting Time

Sets Goal

Completed ?

1 | 2 | 3 | 4 | 5

1 MONDAY

EXERCISE & LEVEL

① ② ③ ④ ⑤

Exercise Time

Resting Time

Sets Goal

Completed ?

1 | 2 | 3 | 4 | 5

2 TUESDAY

EXERCISE & LEVEL

① ② ③ ④ ⑤

Exercise Time

Resting Time

Sets Goal

Completed ?

1 | 2 | 3 | 4 | 5

3 WEDNESDAY

EXERCISE & LEVEL

① ② ③ ④ ⑤

Exercise Time

Resting Time

Sets Goal

Completed ?

1 | 2 | 3 | 4 | 5

4 THURSDAY

EXERCISE & LEVEL

① ② ③ ④ ⑤

Exercise Time

Resting Time

Sets Goal

Completed ?

1 | 2 | 3 | 4 | 5

5 FRIDAY

Move on to the next step if you have completed five ticks in a row. ☑

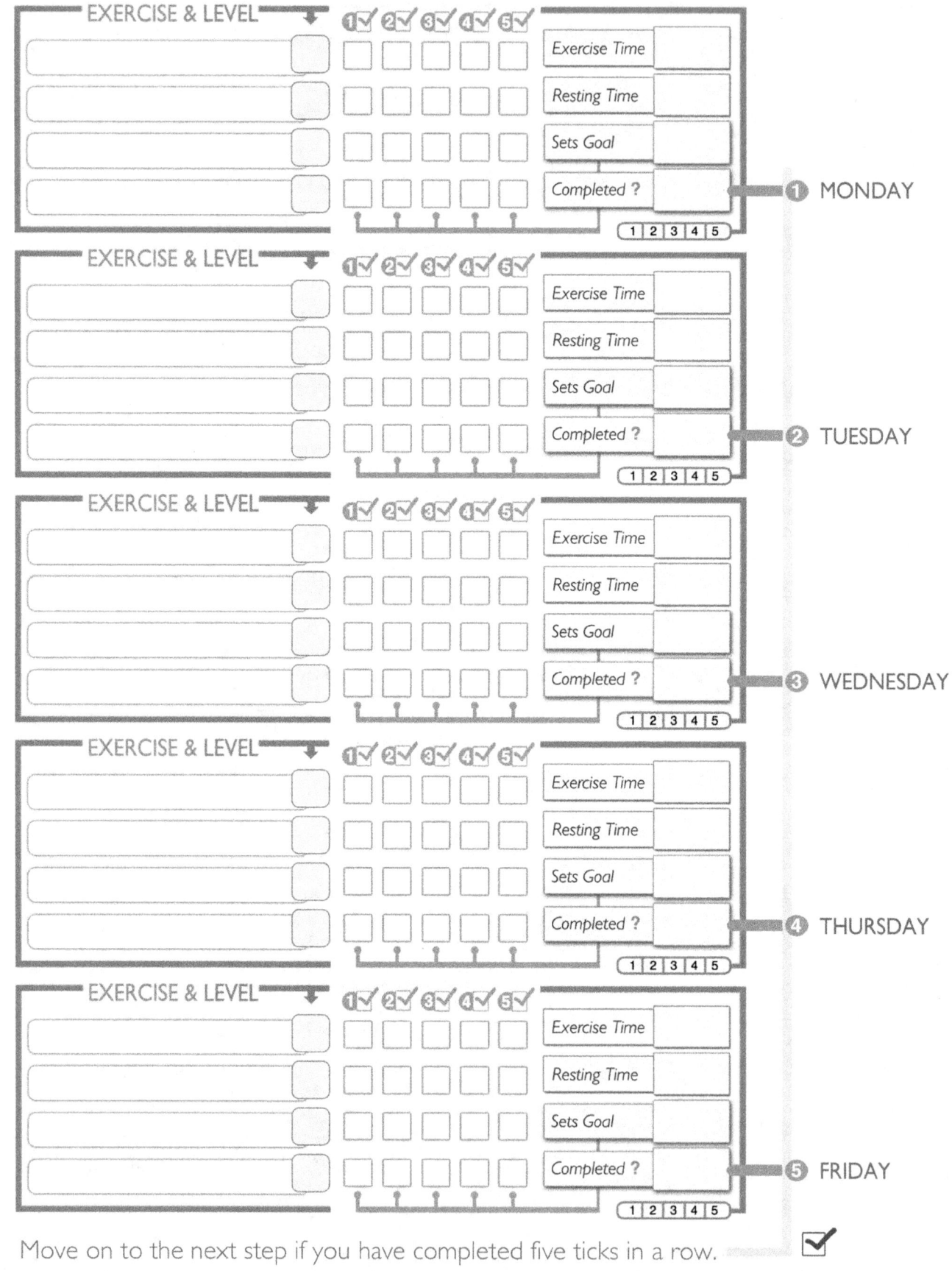

Move on to the next step if you have completed five ticks in a row.

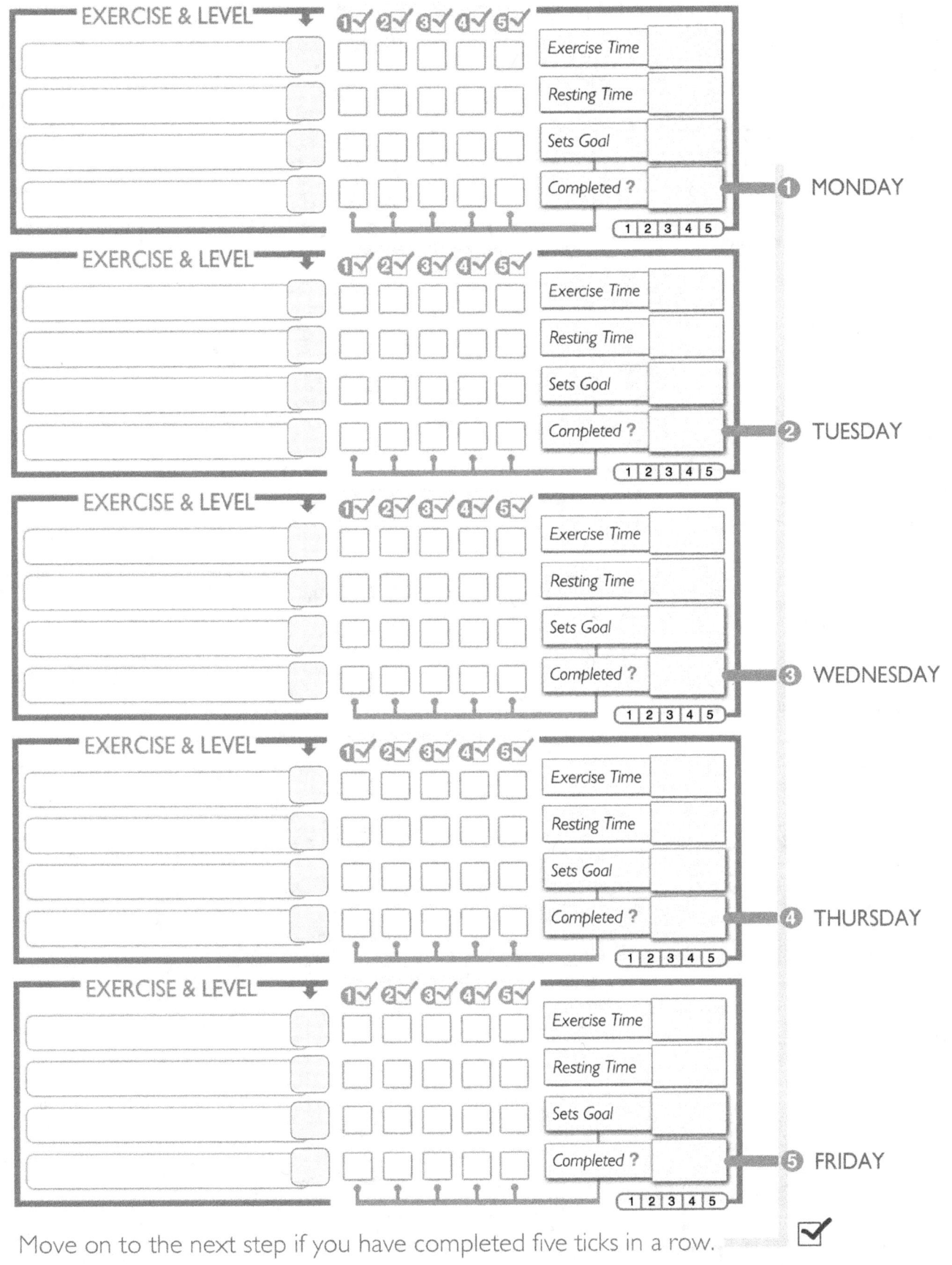

EXERCISE & LEVEL

1 ✓ 2 ✓ 3 ✓ 4 ✓ 5 ✓

Exercise Time

Resting Time

Sets Goal

Completed ?

1 | 2 | 3 | 4 | 5

❶ MONDAY

EXERCISE & LEVEL

1 ✓ 2 ✓ 3 ✓ 4 ✓ 5 ✓

Exercise Time

Resting Time

Sets Goal

Completed ?

1 | 2 | 3 | 4 | 5

❷ TUESDAY

EXERCISE & LEVEL

1 ✓ 2 ✓ 3 ✓ 4 ✓ 5 ✓

Exercise Time

Resting Time

Sets Goal

Completed ?

1 | 2 | 3 | 4 | 5

❸ WEDNESDAY

EXERCISE & LEVEL

1 ✓ 2 ✓ 3 ✓ 4 ✓ 5 ✓

Exercise Time

Resting Time

Sets Goal

Completed ?

1 | 2 | 3 | 4 | 5

❹ THURSDAY

EXERCISE & LEVEL

1 ✓ 2 ✓ 3 ✓ 4 ✓ 5 ✓

Exercise Time

Resting Time

Sets Goal

Completed ?

1 | 2 | 3 | 4 | 5

❺ FRIDAY

Move on to the next step if you have completed five ticks in a row. ☑

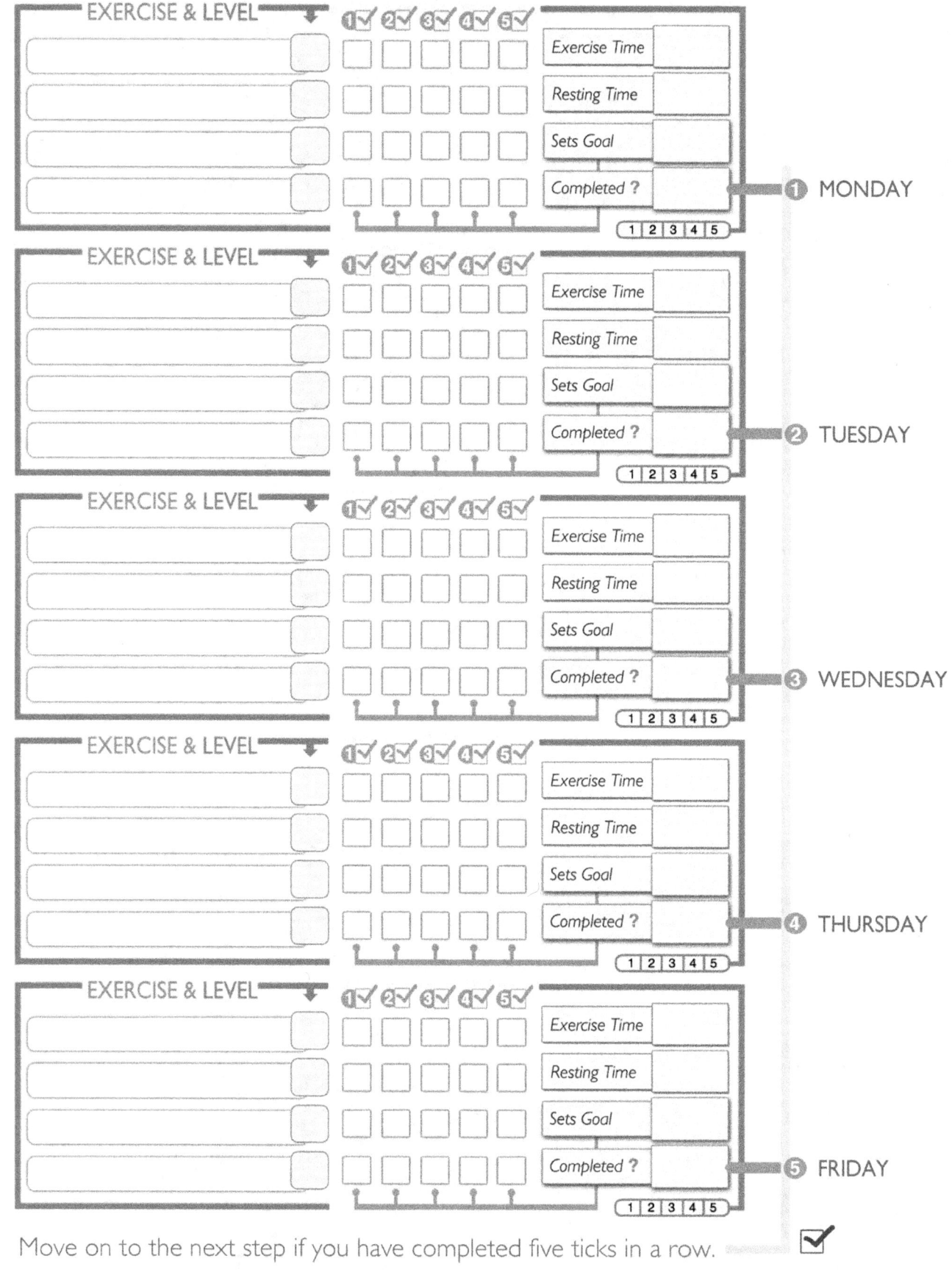

EXERCISE & LEVEL ①✓ ②✓ ③✓ ④✓ ⑤✓

Exercise Time

Resting Time

Sets Goal

Completed ?

❶ MONDAY

1 2 3 4 5

EXERCISE & LEVEL ①✓ ②✓ ③✓ ④✓ ⑤✓

Exercise Time

Resting Time

Sets Goal

Completed ?

❷ TUESDAY

1 2 3 4 5

EXERCISE & LEVEL ①✓ ②✓ ③✓ ④✓ ⑤✓

Exercise Time

Resting Time

Sets Goal

Completed ?

❸ WEDNESDAY

1 2 3 4 5

EXERCISE & LEVEL ①✓ ②✓ ③✓ ④✓ ⑤✓

Exercise Time

Resting Time

Sets Goal

Completed ?

❹ THURSDAY

1 2 3 4 5

EXERCISE & LEVEL ①✓ ②✓ ③✓ ④✓ ⑤✓

Exercise Time

Resting Time

Sets Goal

Completed ?

❺ FRIDAY

1 2 3 4 5

Move on to the next step if you have completed five ticks in a row. ✓

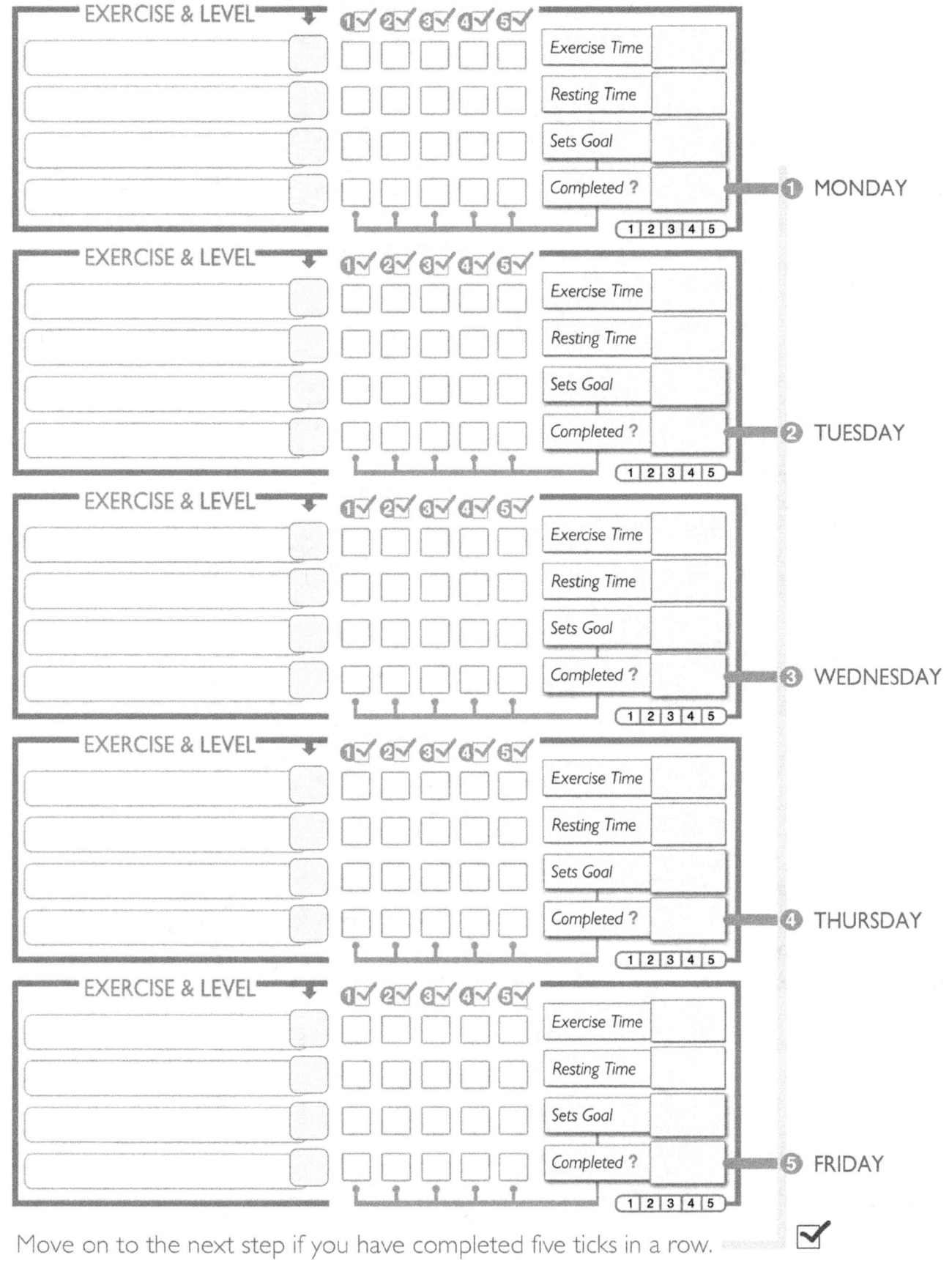

Move on to the next step if you have completed five ticks in a row.

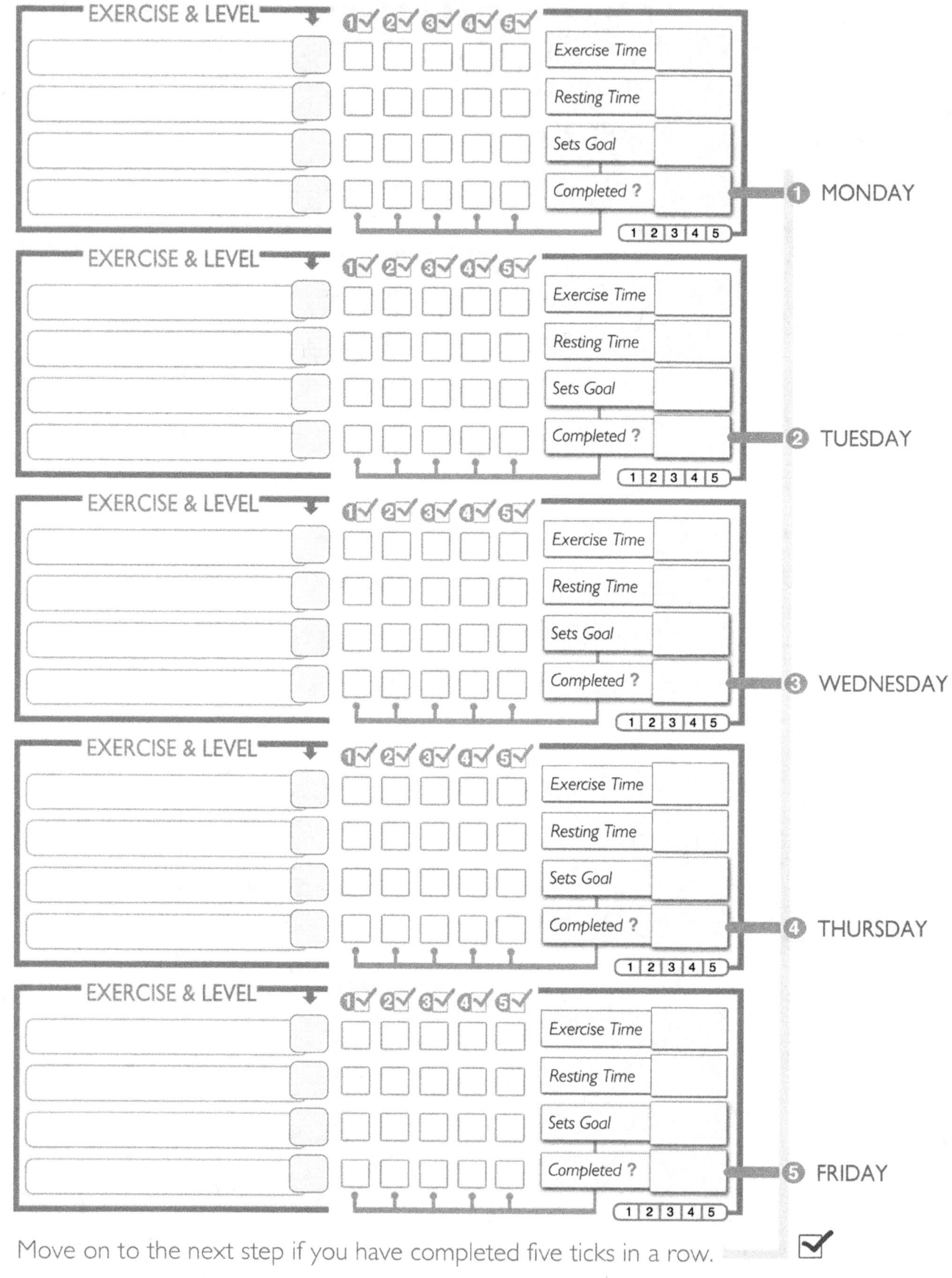

Move on to the next step if you have completed five ticks in a row.

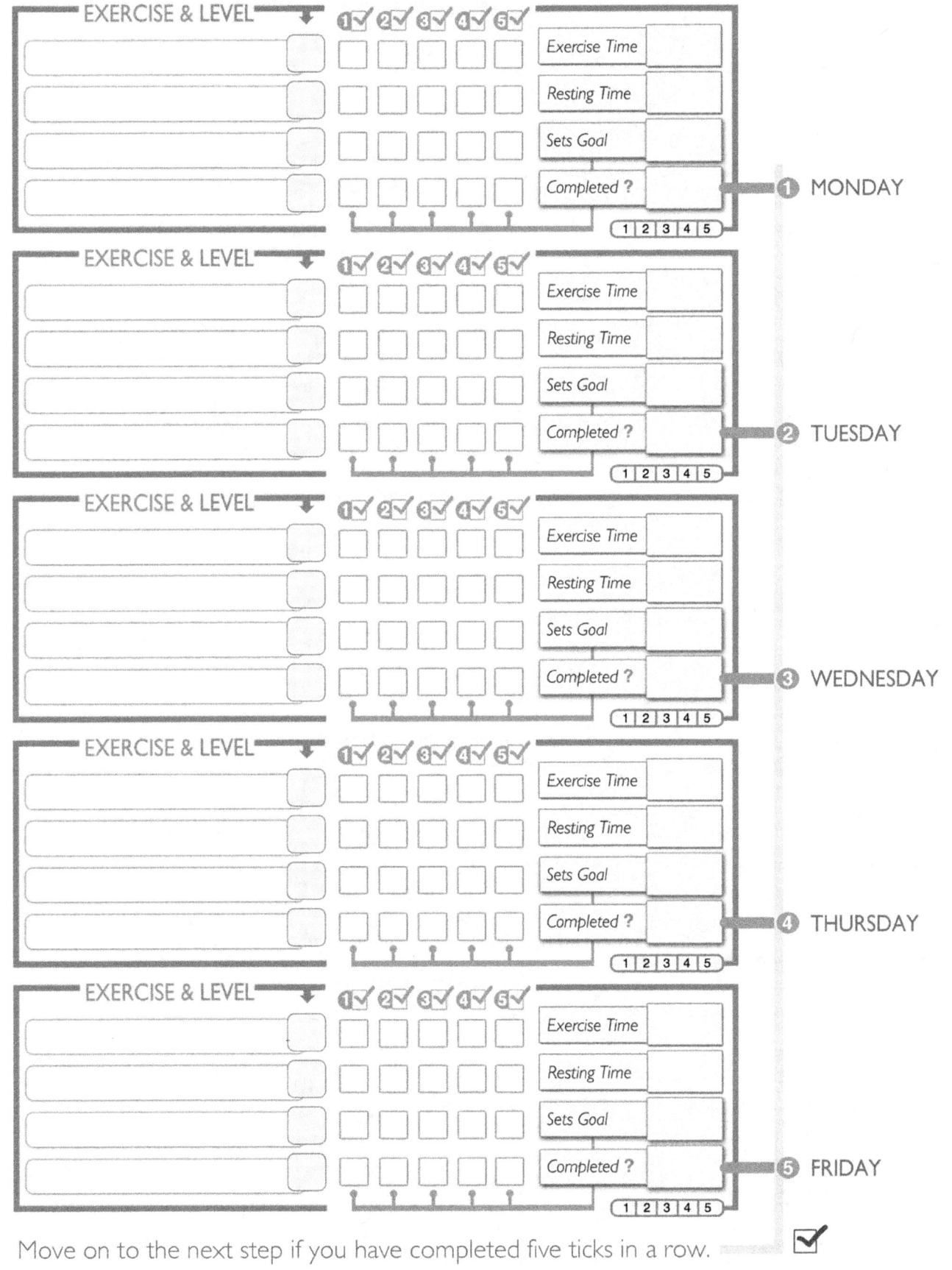

Move on to the next step if you have completed five ticks in a row.

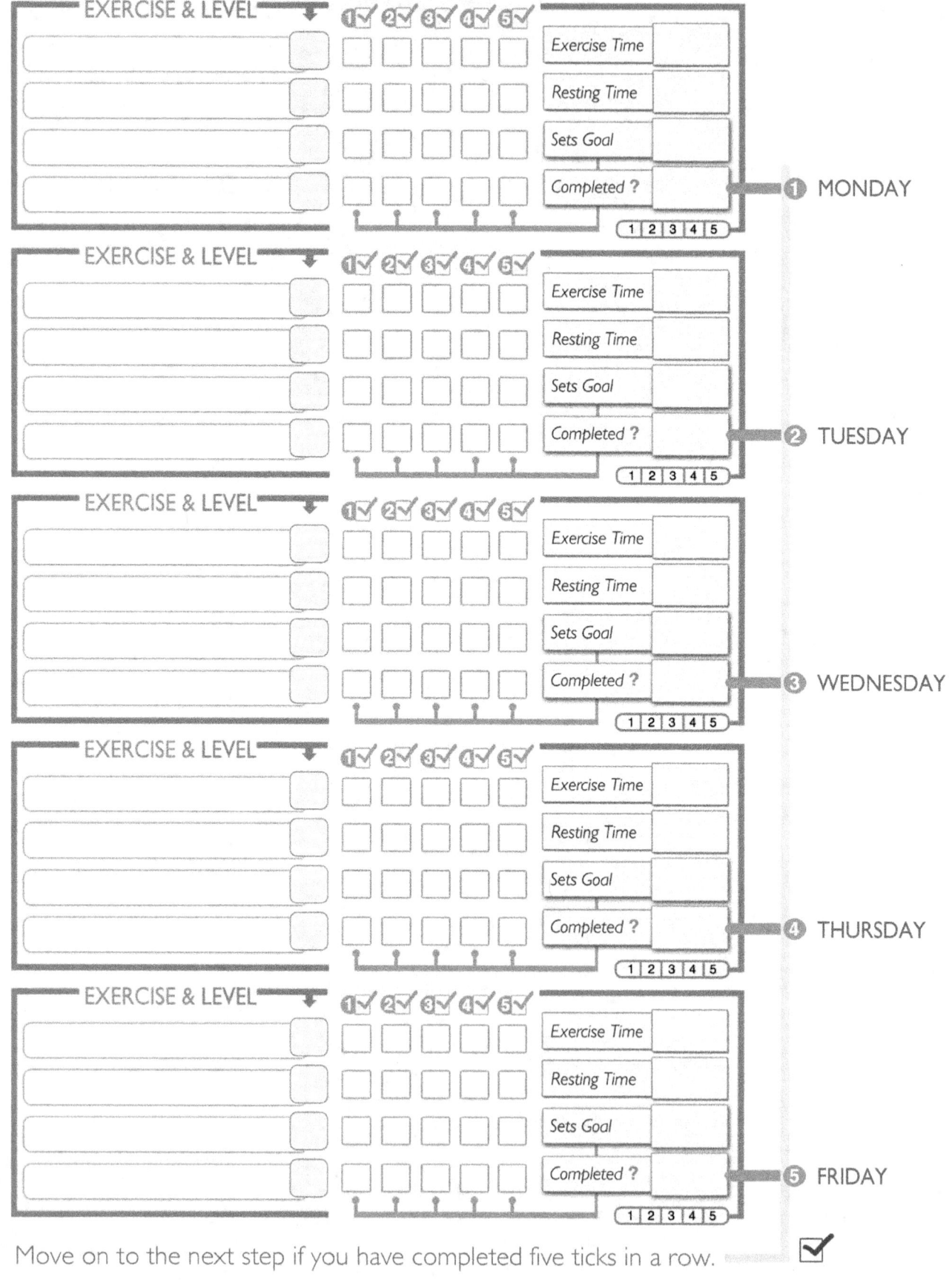

EXERCISE & LEVEL — 1✓ 2✓ 3✓ 4✓ 5✓

Exercise Time
Resting Time
Sets Goal
Completed ?

1 2 3 4 5

① MONDAY

EXERCISE & LEVEL — 1✓ 2✓ 3✓ 4✓ 5✓

Exercise Time
Resting Time
Sets Goal
Completed ?

1 2 3 4 5

② TUESDAY

EXERCISE & LEVEL — 1✓ 2✓ 3✓ 4✓ 5✓

Exercise Time
Resting Time
Sets Goal
Completed ?

1 2 3 4 5

③ WEDNESDAY

EXERCISE & LEVEL — 1✓ 2✓ 3✓ 4✓ 5✓

Exercise Time
Resting Time
Sets Goal
Completed ?

1 2 3 4 5

④ THURSDAY

EXERCISE & LEVEL — 1✓ 2✓ 3✓ 4✓ 5✓

Exercise Time
Resting Time
Sets Goal
Completed ?

1 2 3 4 5

⑤ FRIDAY

Move on to the next step if you have completed five ticks in a row. ✓

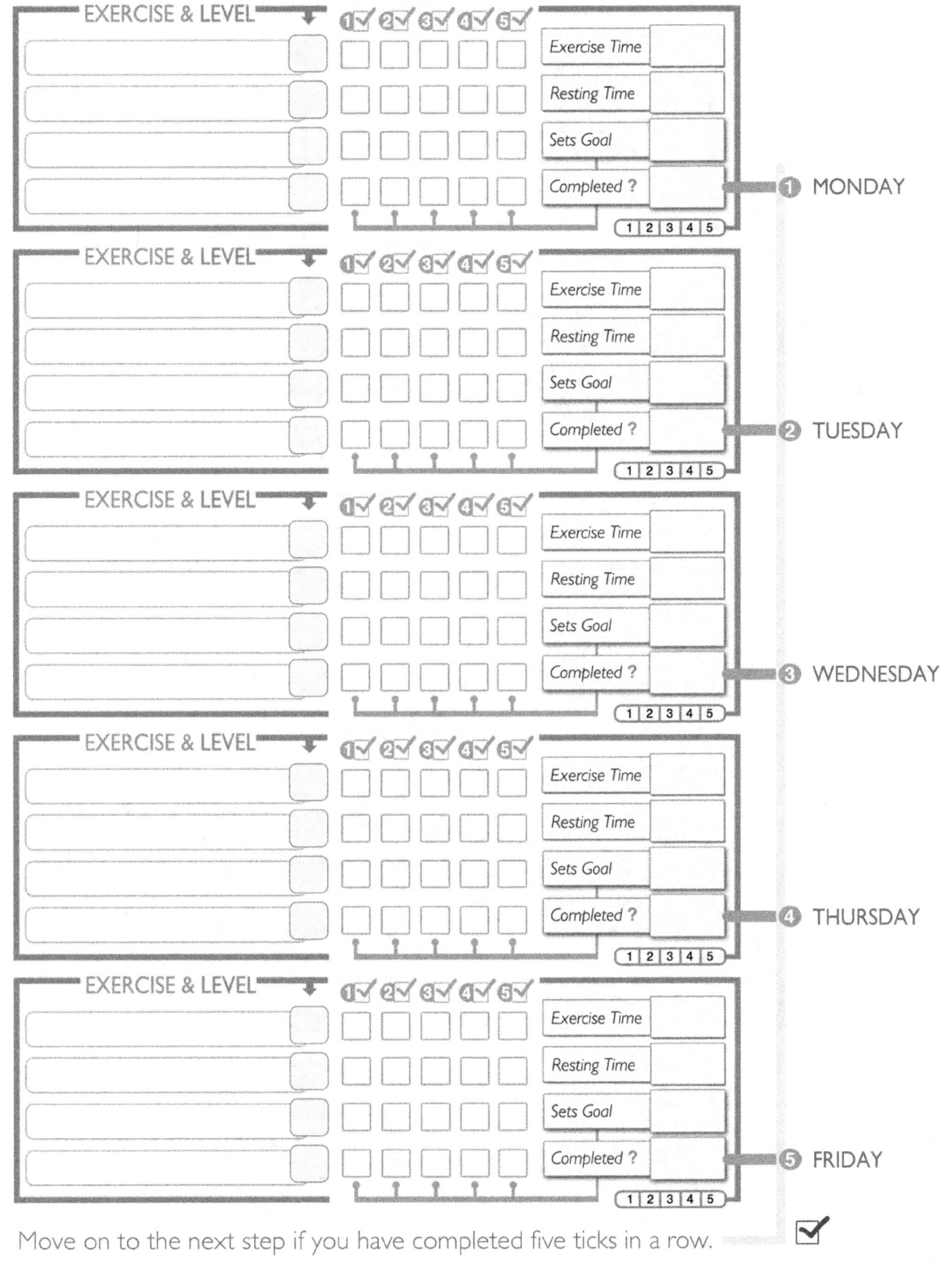

EXERCISE & LEVEL ① ② ③ ④ ⑤

Exercise Time
Resting Time
Sets Goal
Completed ?

1 MONDAY

1 2 3 4 5

EXERCISE & LEVEL ① ② ③ ④ ⑤

Exercise Time
Resting Time
Sets Goal
Completed ?

2 TUESDAY

1 2 3 4 5

EXERCISE & LEVEL ① ② ③ ④ ⑤

Exercise Time
Resting Time
Sets Goal
Completed ?

3 WEDNESDAY

1 2 3 4 5

EXERCISE & LEVEL ① ② ③ ④ ⑤

Exercise Time
Resting Time
Sets Goal
Completed ?

4 THURSDAY

1 2 3 4 5

EXERCISE & LEVEL ① ② ③ ④ ⑤

Exercise Time
Resting Time
Sets Goal
Completed ?

5 FRIDAY

1 2 3 4 5

Move on to the next step if you have completed five ticks in a row.

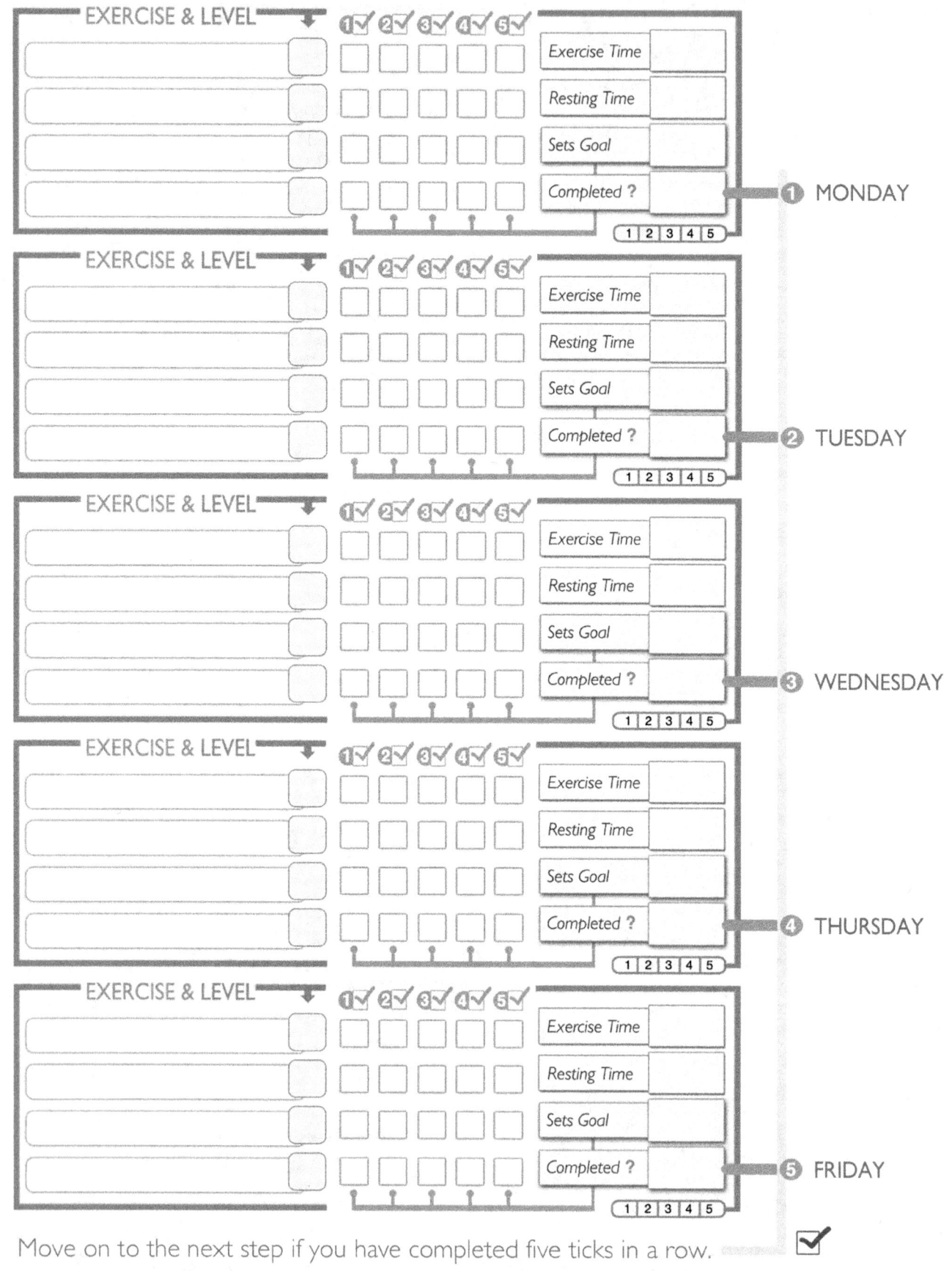

EXERCISE & LEVEL ✓

| 1 ✓ | 2 ✓ | 3 ✓ | 4 ✓ | 5 ✓ |

Exercise Time

Resting Time

Sets Goal

Completed ?

1 2 3 4 5

❶ MONDAY

EXERCISE & LEVEL ✓

| 1 ✓ | 2 ✓ | 3 ✓ | 4 ✓ | 5 ✓ |

Exercise Time

Resting Time

Sets Goal

Completed ?

1 2 3 4 5

❷ TUESDAY

EXERCISE & LEVEL ✓

| 1 ✓ | 2 ✓ | 3 ✓ | 4 ✓ | 5 ✓ |

Exercise Time

Resting Time

Sets Goal

Completed ?

1 2 3 4 5

❸ WEDNESDAY

EXERCISE & LEVEL ✓

| 1 ✓ | 2 ✓ | 3 ✓ | 4 ✓ | 5 ✓ |

Exercise Time

Resting Time

Sets Goal

Completed ?

1 2 3 4 5

❹ THURSDAY

EXERCISE & LEVEL ✓

| 1 ✓ | 2 ✓ | 3 ✓ | 4 ✓ | 5 ✓ |

Exercise Time

Resting Time

Sets Goal

Completed ?

1 2 3 4 5

❺ FRIDAY

Move on to the next step if you have completed five ticks in a row. ✓

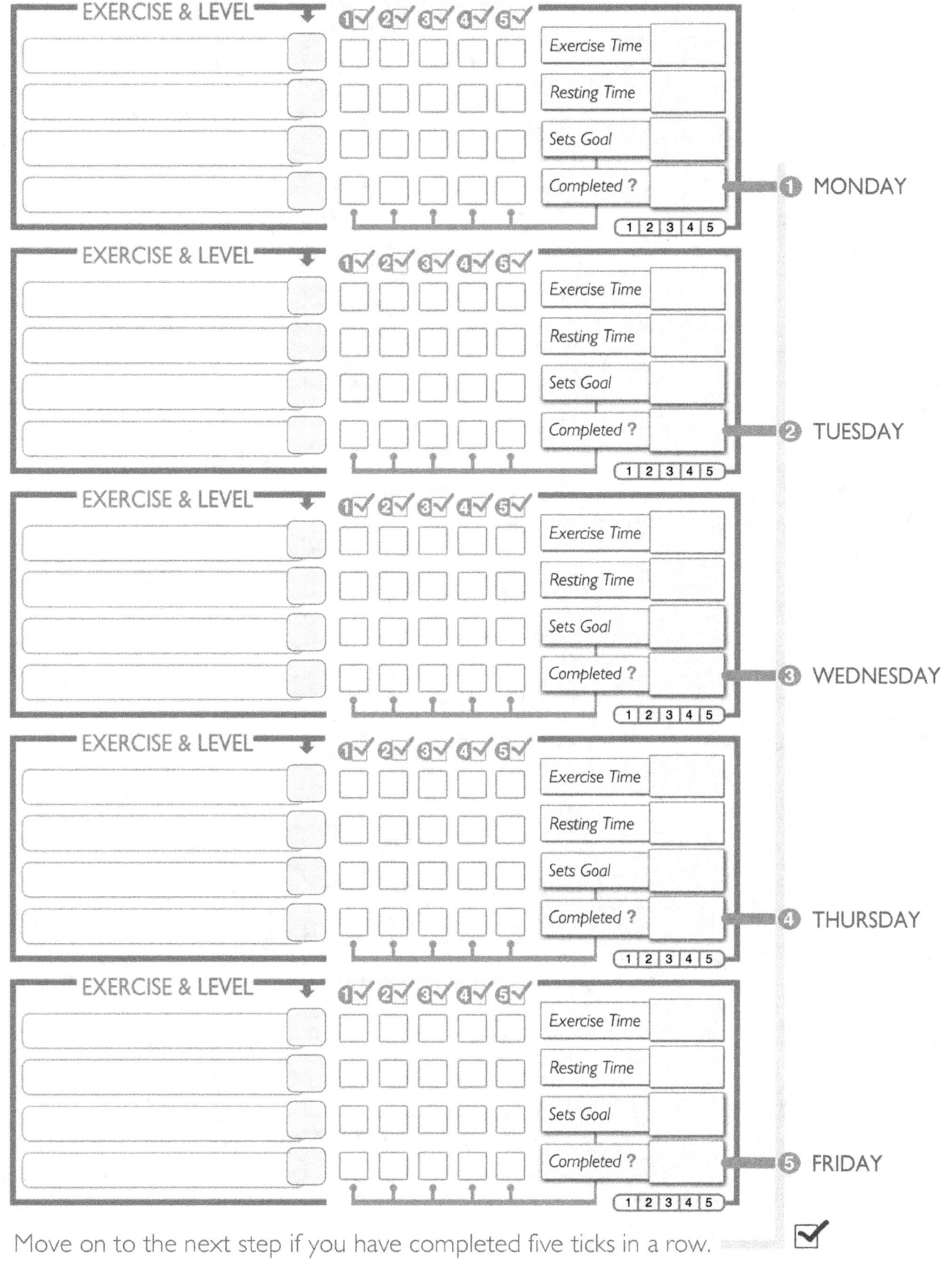

EXERCISE & LEVEL ▼ 1☑ 2☑ 3☑ 4☑ 5☑

Exercise Time
Resting Time
Sets Goal
Completed ?

1 MONDAY

1 2 3 4 5

EXERCISE & LEVEL ▼ 1☑ 2☑ 3☑ 4☑ 5☑

Exercise Time
Resting Time
Sets Goal
Completed ?

2 TUESDAY

1 2 3 4 5

EXERCISE & LEVEL ▼ 1☑ 2☑ 3☑ 4☑ 5☑

Exercise Time
Resting Time
Sets Goal
Completed ?

3 WEDNESDAY

1 2 3 4 5

EXERCISE & LEVEL ▼ 1☑ 2☑ 3☑ 4☑ 5☑

Exercise Time
Resting Time
Sets Goal
Completed ?

4 THURSDAY

1 2 3 4 5

EXERCISE & LEVEL ▼ 1☑ 2☑ 3☑ 4☑ 5☑

Exercise Time
Resting Time
Sets Goal
Completed ?

5 FRIDAY

1 2 3 4 5

Move on to the next step if you have completed five ticks in a row. ☑

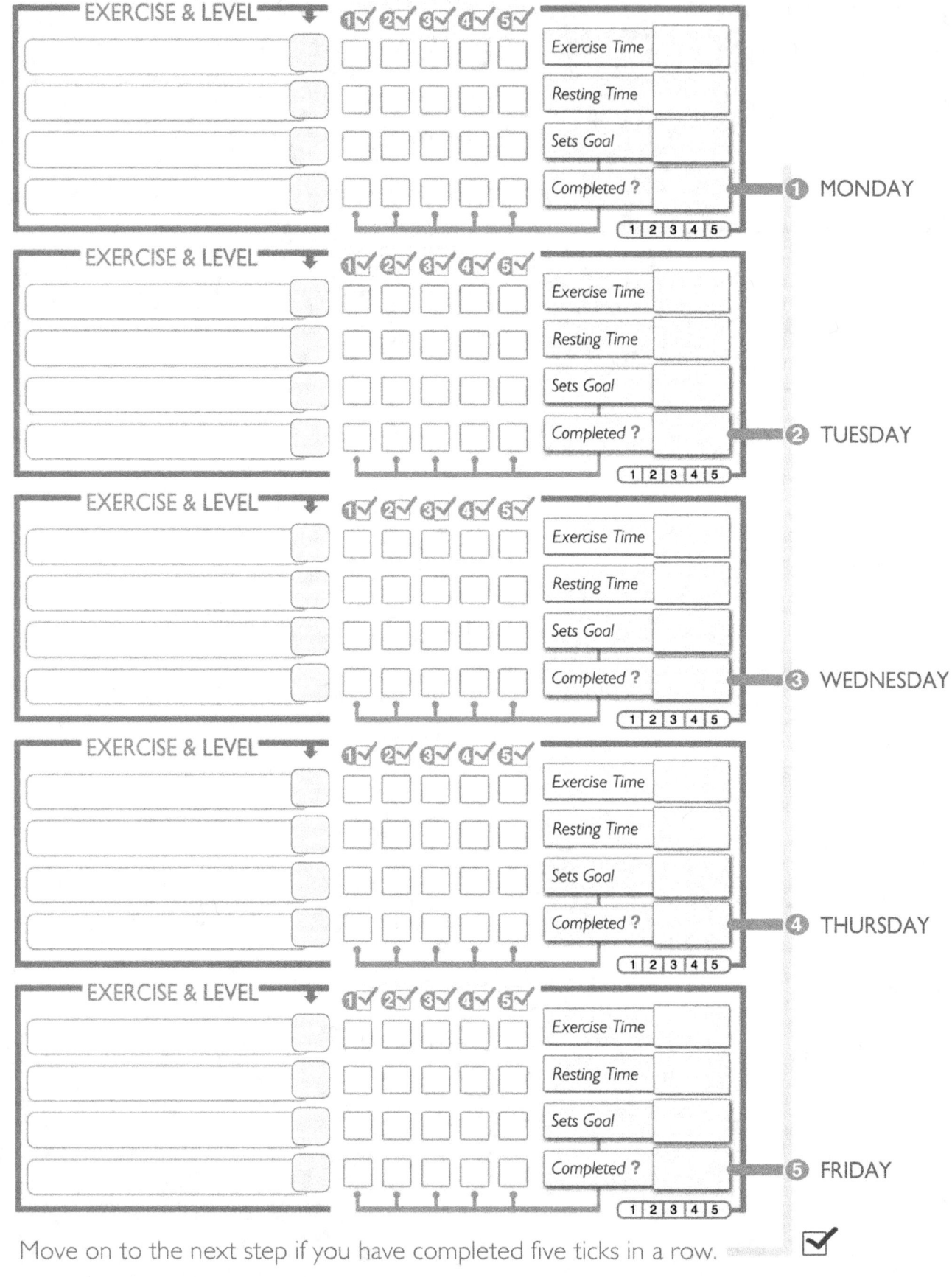

EXERCISE & LEVEL   ✓1 ✓2 ✓3 ✓4 ✓5

Exercise Time
Resting Time
Sets Goal
Completed ?   ❶ MONDAY
1 2 3 4 5

EXERCISE & LEVEL   ✓1 ✓2 ✓3 ✓4 ✓5

Exercise Time
Resting Time
Sets Goal
Completed ?   ❷ TUESDAY
1 2 3 4 5

EXERCISE & LEVEL   ✓1 ✓2 ✓3 ✓4 ✓5

Exercise Time
Resting Time
Sets Goal
Completed ?   ❸ WEDNESDAY
1 2 3 4 5

EXERCISE & LEVEL   ✓1 ✓2 ✓3 ✓4 ✓5

Exercise Time
Resting Time
Sets Goal
Completed ?   ❹ THURSDAY
1 2 3 4 5

EXERCISE & LEVEL   ✓1 ✓2 ✓3 ✓4 ✓5

Exercise Time
Resting Time
Sets Goal
Completed ?   ❺ FRIDAY
1 2 3 4 5

Move on to the next step if you have completed five ticks in a row. ☑

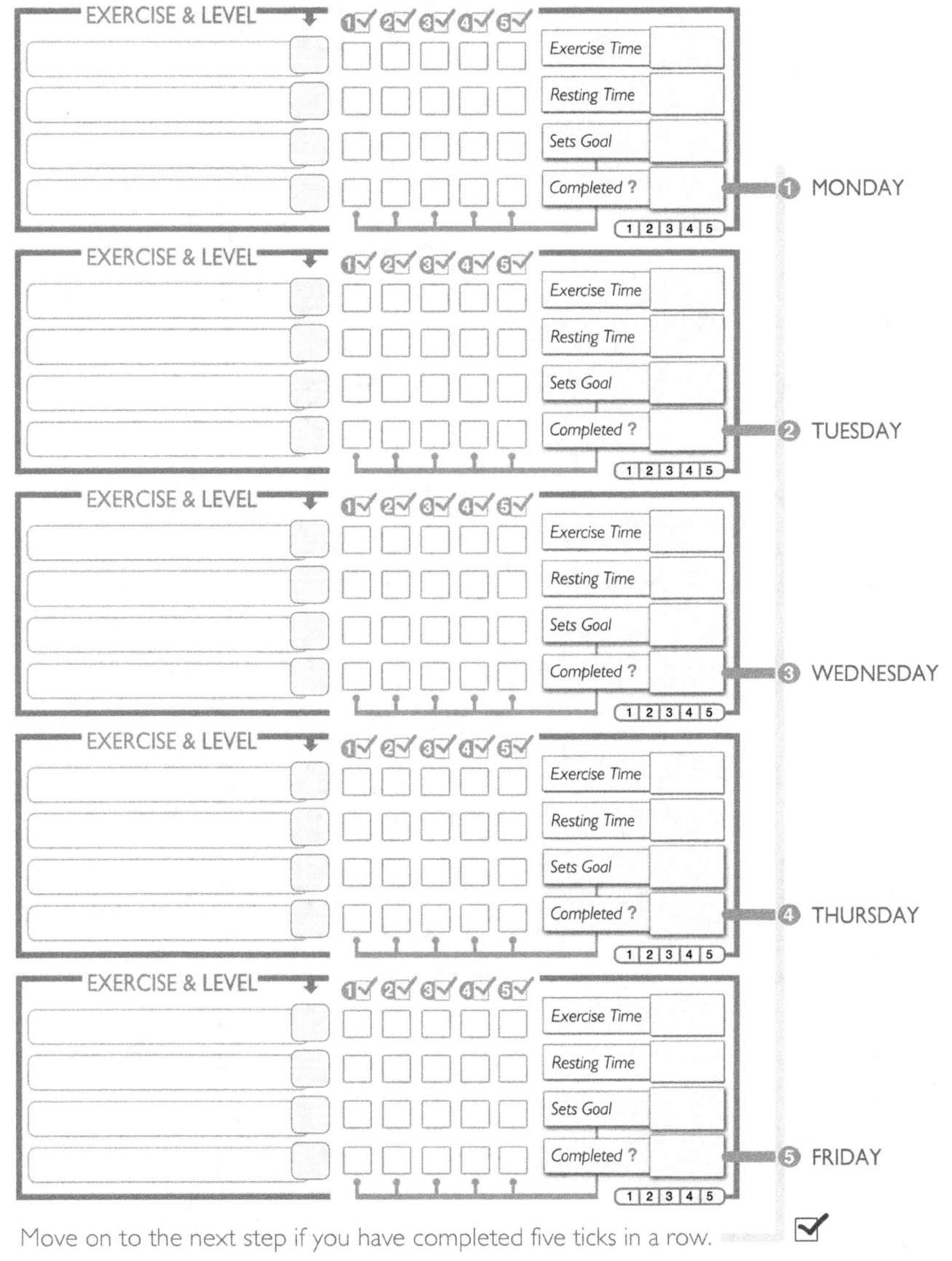

EXERCISE & LEVEL

1☑ 2☑ 3☑ 4☑ 5☑

Exercise Time
Resting Time
Sets Goal
Completed ?

❶ MONDAY

1 2 3 4 5

EXERCISE & LEVEL

1☑ 2☑ 3☑ 4☑ 5☑

Exercise Time
Resting Time
Sets Goal
Completed ?

❷ TUESDAY

1 2 3 4 5

EXERCISE & LEVEL

1☑ 2☑ 3☑ 4☑ 5☑

Exercise Time
Resting Time
Sets Goal
Completed ?

❸ WEDNESDAY

1 2 3 4 5

EXERCISE & LEVEL

1☑ 2☑ 3☑ 4☑ 5☑

Exercise Time
Resting Time
Sets Goal
Completed ?

❹ THURSDAY

1 2 3 4 5

EXERCISE & LEVEL

1☑ 2☑ 3☑ 4☑ 5☑

Exercise Time
Resting Time
Sets Goal
Completed ?

❺ FRIDAY

1 2 3 4 5

Move on to the next step if you have completed five ticks in a row. ☑

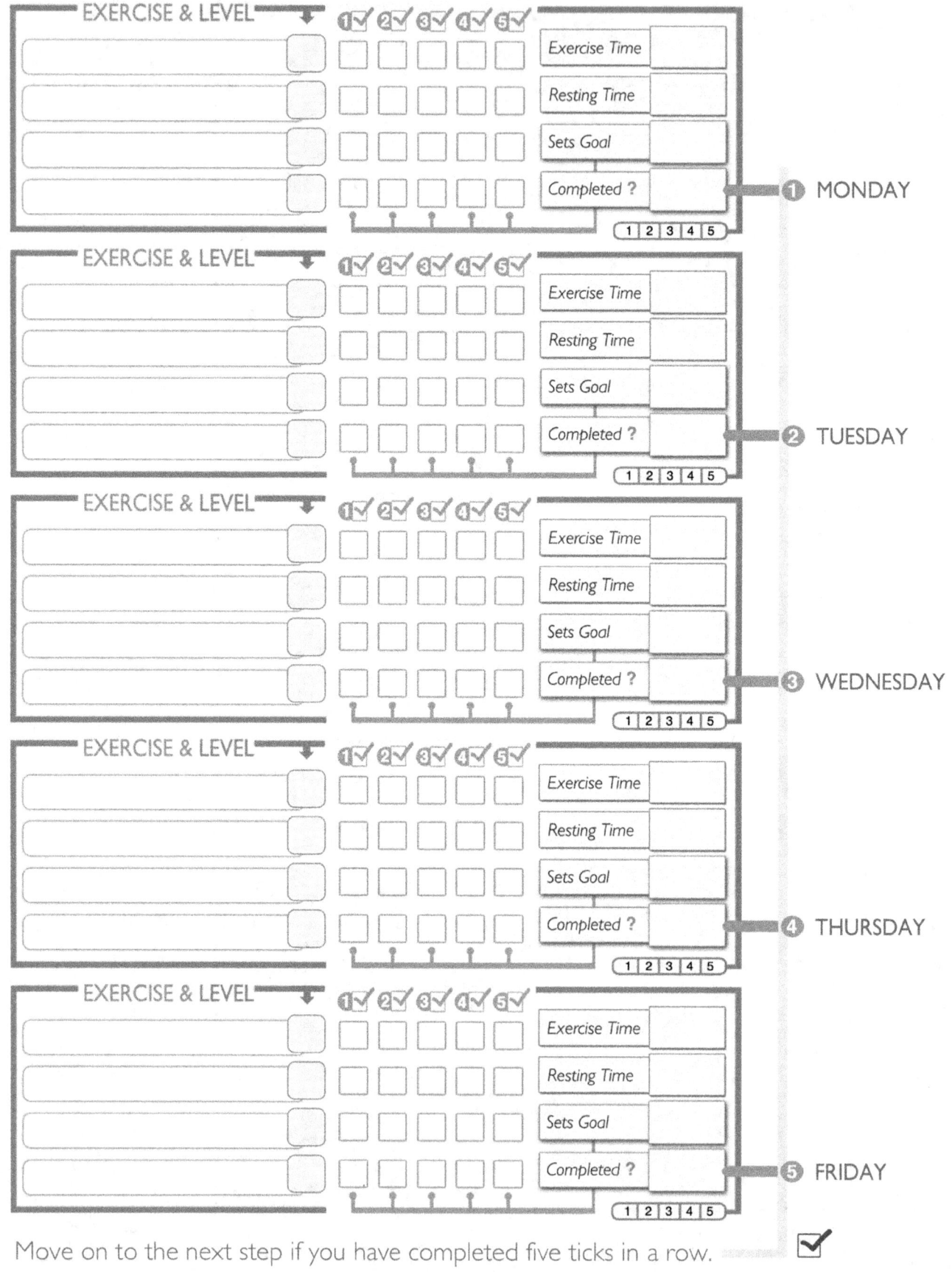

EXERCISE & LEVEL   1✓ 2✓ 3✓ 4✓ 5✓

Exercise Time

Resting Time

Sets Goal

Completed ?

1 2 3 4 5

1 MONDAY

EXERCISE & LEVEL   1✓ 2✓ 3✓ 4✓ 5✓

Exercise Time

Resting Time

Sets Goal

Completed ?

1 2 3 4 5

2 TUESDAY

EXERCISE & LEVEL   1✓ 2✓ 3✓ 4✓ 5✓

Exercise Time

Resting Time

Sets Goal

Completed ?

1 2 3 4 5

3 WEDNESDAY

EXERCISE & LEVEL   1✓ 2✓ 3✓ 4✓ 5✓

Exercise Time

Resting Time

Sets Goal

Completed ?

1 2 3 4 5

4 THURSDAY

EXERCISE & LEVEL   1✓ 2✓ 3✓ 4✓ 5✓

Exercise Time

Resting Time

Sets Goal

Completed ?

1 2 3 4 5

5 FRIDAY

Move on to the next step if you have completed five ticks in a row. ✓

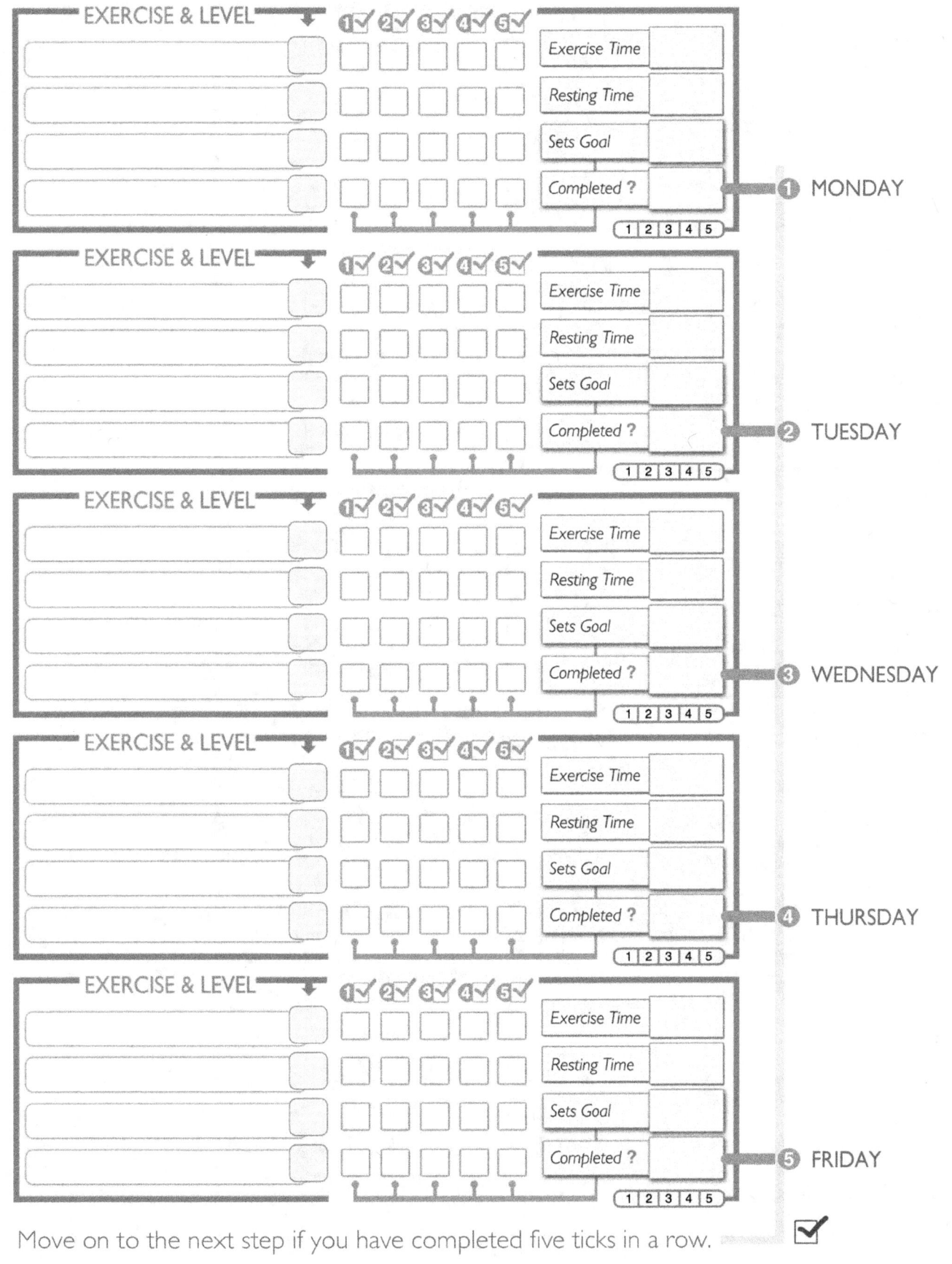

EXERCISE & LEVEL

1✓ 2✓ 3✓ 4✓ 5✓

Exercise Time
Resting Time
Sets Goal
Completed ?

1 | 2 | 3 | 4 | 5

❶ MONDAY

EXERCISE & LEVEL

1✓ 2✓ 3✓ 4✓ 5✓

Exercise Time
Resting Time
Sets Goal
Completed ?

1 | 2 | 3 | 4 | 5

❷ TUESDAY

EXERCISE & LEVEL

1✓ 2✓ 3✓ 4✓ 5✓

Exercise Time
Resting Time
Sets Goal
Completed ?

1 | 2 | 3 | 4 | 5

❸ WEDNESDAY

EXERCISE & LEVEL

1✓ 2✓ 3✓ 4✓ 5✓

Exercise Time
Resting Time
Sets Goal
Completed ?

1 | 2 | 3 | 4 | 5

❹ THURSDAY

EXERCISE & LEVEL

1✓ 2✓ 3✓ 4✓ 5✓

Exercise Time
Resting Time
Sets Goal
Completed ?

1 | 2 | 3 | 4 | 5

❺ FRIDAY

Move on to the next step if you have completed five ticks in a row. ✓

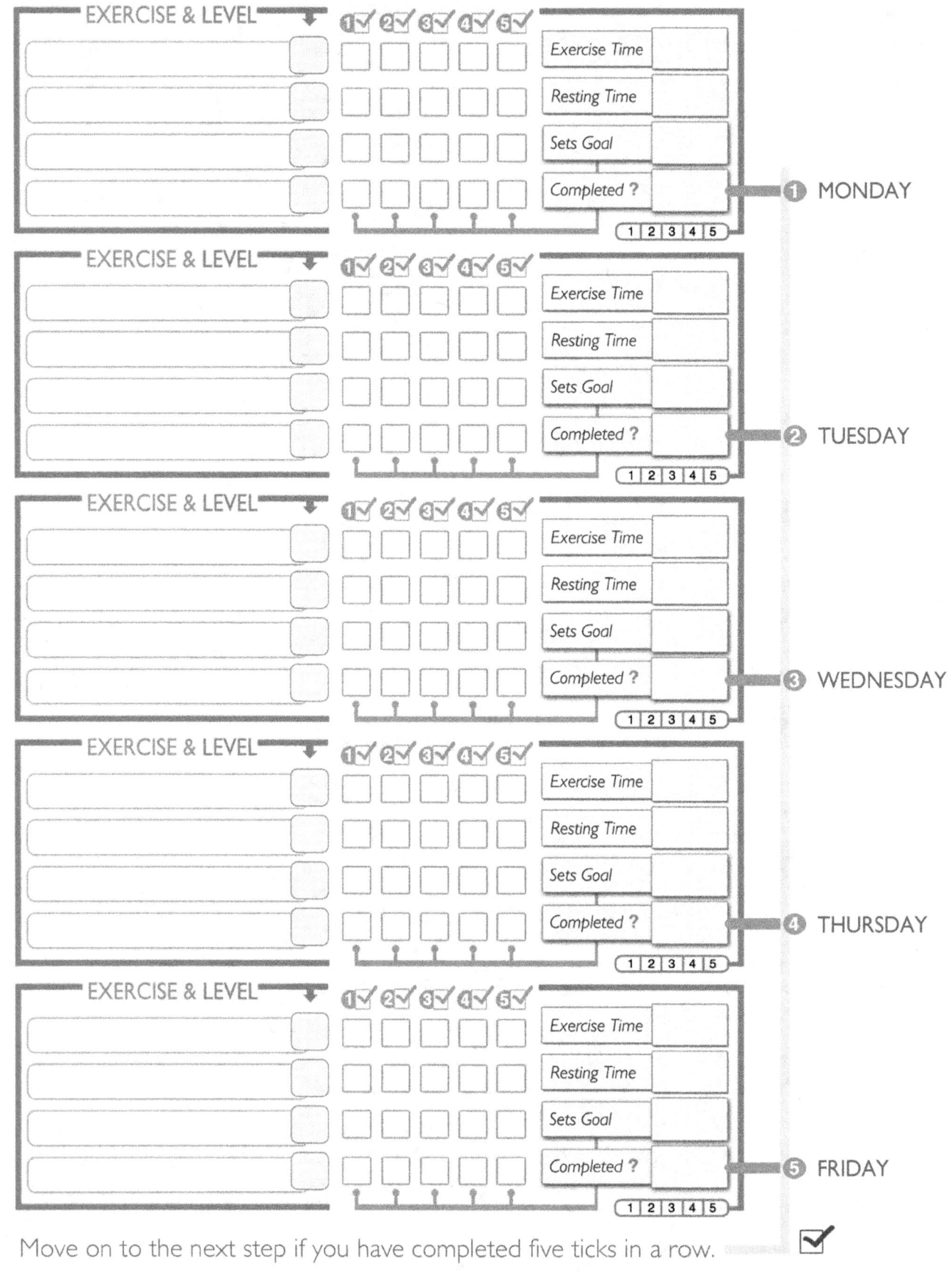

Move on to the next step if you have completed five ticks in a row.

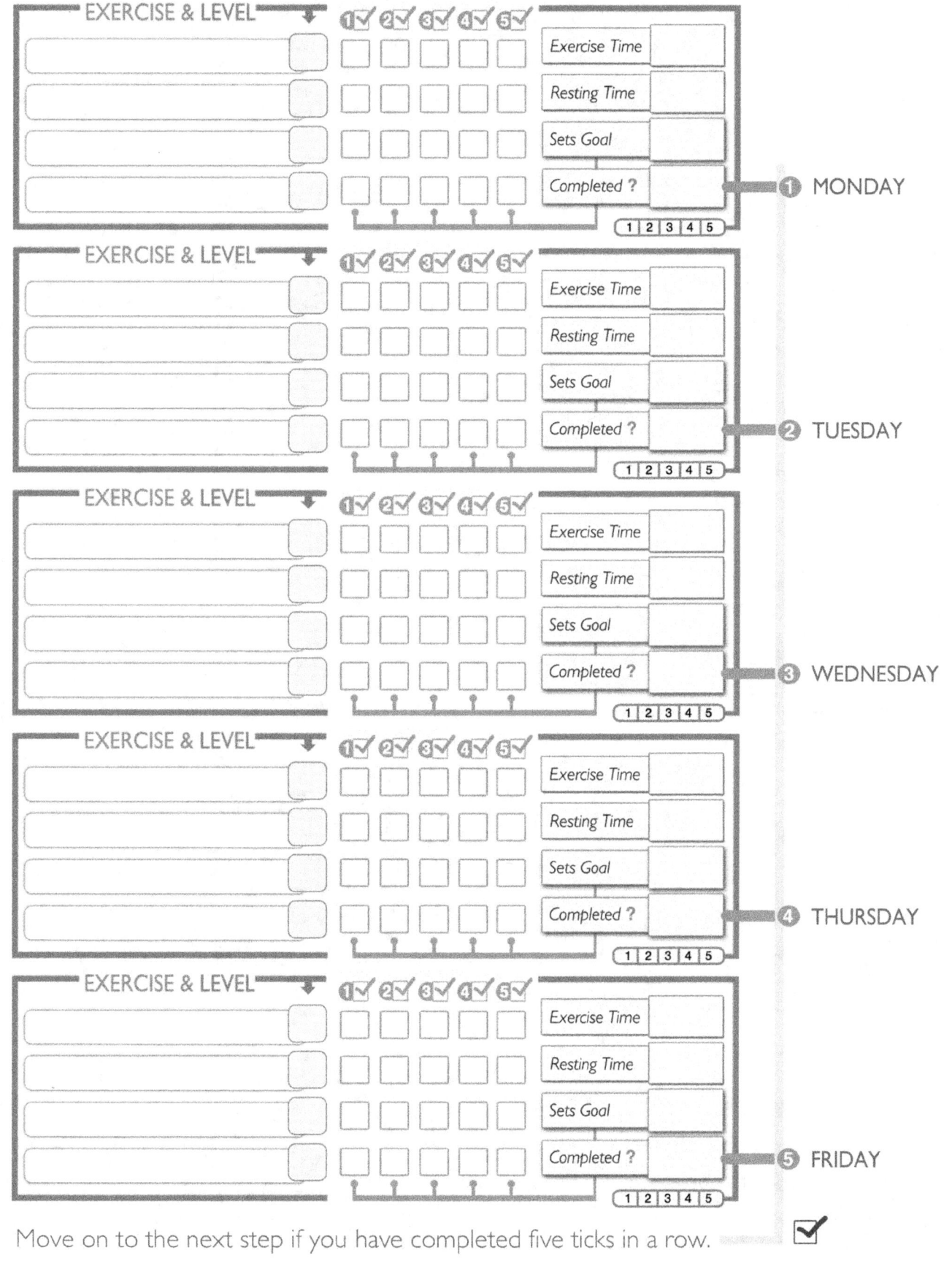

EXERCISE & LEVEL ▼ 1✓ 2✓ 3✓ 4✓ 5✓

Exercise Time
Resting Time
Sets Goal
Completed ?

❶ MONDAY

1 2 3 4 5

EXERCISE & LEVEL ▼ 1✓ 2✓ 3✓ 4✓ 5✓

Exercise Time
Resting Time
Sets Goal
Completed ?

❷ TUESDAY

1 2 3 4 5

EXERCISE & LEVEL ▼ 1✓ 2✓ 3✓ 4✓ 5✓

Exercise Time
Resting Time
Sets Goal
Completed ?

❸ WEDNESDAY

1 2 3 4 5

EXERCISE & LEVEL ▼ 1✓ 2✓ 3✓ 4✓ 5✓

Exercise Time
Resting Time
Sets Goal
Completed ?

❹ THURSDAY

1 2 3 4 5

EXERCISE & LEVEL ▼ 1✓ 2✓ 3✓ 4✓ 5✓

Exercise Time
Resting Time
Sets Goal
Completed ?

❺ FRIDAY

1 2 3 4 5

Move on to the next step if you have completed five ticks in a row. ✓

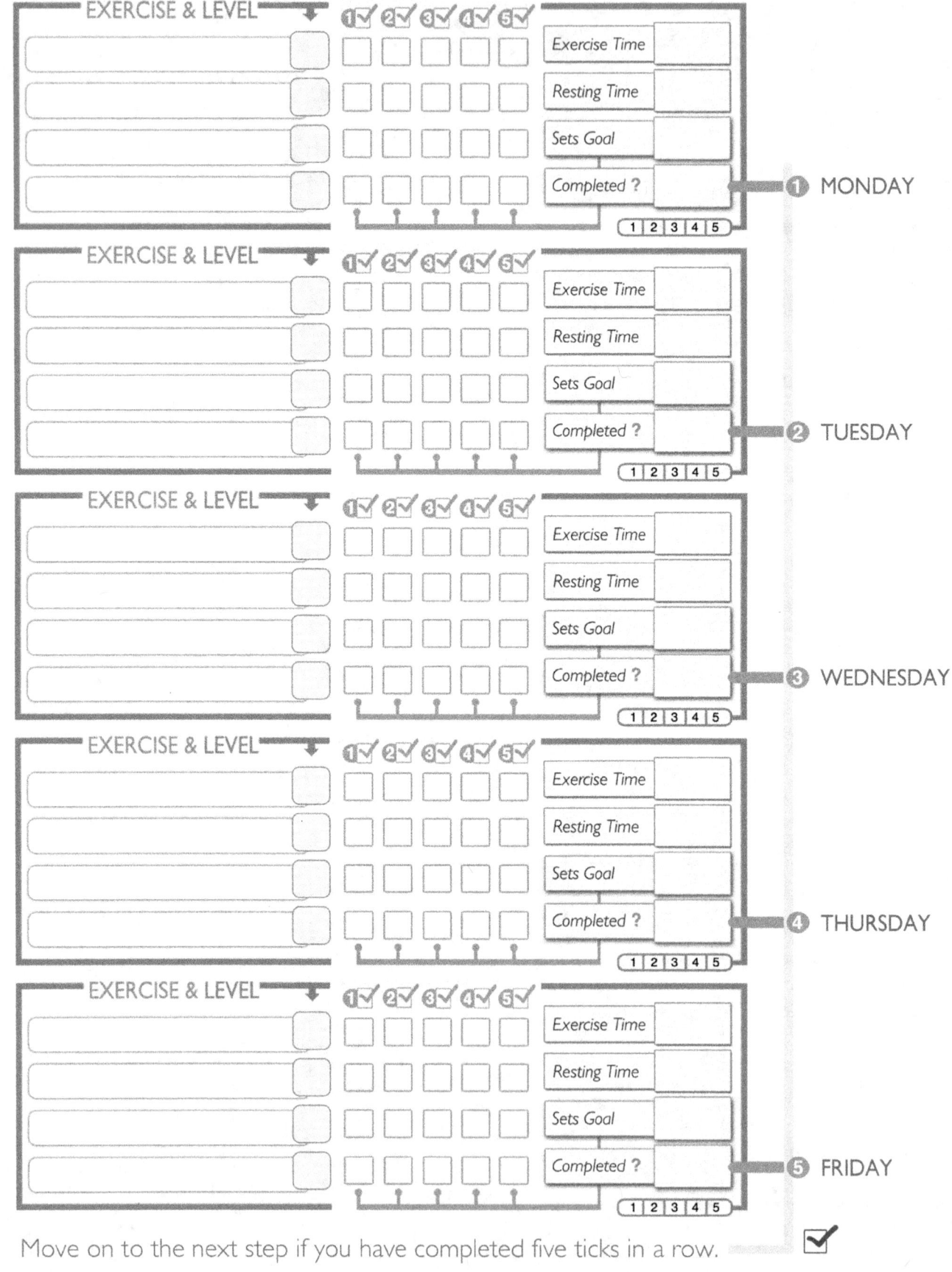

EXERCISE & LEVEL   1✓ 2✓ 3✓ 4✓ 5✓

Exercise Time

Resting Time

Sets Goal

Completed ?   1 2 3 4 5

① MONDAY

EXERCISE & LEVEL   1✓ 2✓ 3✓ 4✓ 5✓

Exercise Time

Resting Time

Sets Goal

Completed ?   1 2 3 4 5

② TUESDAY

EXERCISE & LEVEL   1✓ 2✓ 3✓ 4✓ 5✓

Exercise Time

Resting Time

Sets Goal

Completed ?   1 2 3 4 5

③ WEDNESDAY

EXERCISE & LEVEL   1✓ 2✓ 3✓ 4✓ 5✓

Exercise Time

Resting Time

Sets Goal

Completed ?   1 2 3 4 5

④ THURSDAY

EXERCISE & LEVEL   1✓ 2✓ 3✓ 4✓ 5✓

Exercise Time

Resting Time

Sets Goal

Completed ?   1 2 3 4 5

⑤ FRIDAY

Move on to the next step if you have completed five ticks in a row.   ✓

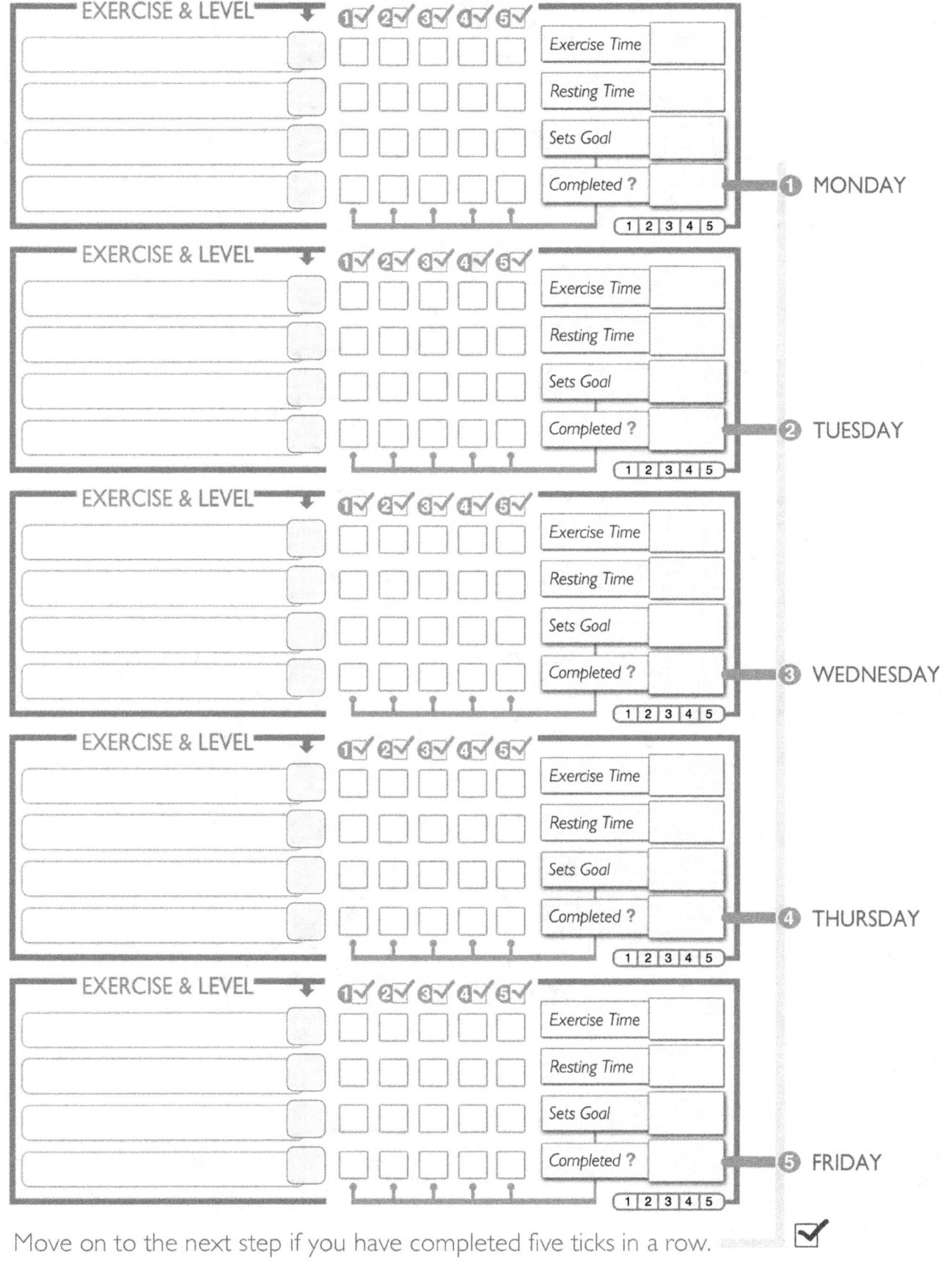

EXERCISE & LEVEL

| 1 ✓ | 2 ✓ | 3 ✓ | 4 ✓ | 5 ✓ |

Exercise Time

Resting Time

Sets Goal

Completed ?

1 2 3 4 5

1 MONDAY

EXERCISE & LEVEL

| 1 ✓ | 2 ✓ | 3 ✓ | 4 ✓ | 5 ✓ |

Exercise Time

Resting Time

Sets Goal

Completed ?

1 2 3 4 5

2 TUESDAY

EXERCISE & LEVEL

| 1 ✓ | 2 ✓ | 3 ✓ | 4 ✓ | 5 ✓ |

Exercise Time

Resting Time

Sets Goal

Completed ?

1 2 3 4 5

3 WEDNESDAY

EXERCISE & LEVEL

| 1 ✓ | 2 ✓ | 3 ✓ | 4 ✓ | 5 ✓ |

Exercise Time

Resting Time

Sets Goal

Completed ?

1 2 3 4 5

4 THURSDAY

EXERCISE & LEVEL

| 1 ✓ | 2 ✓ | 3 ✓ | 4 ✓ | 5 ✓ |

Exercise Time

Resting Time

Sets Goal

Completed ?

1 2 3 4 5

5 FRIDAY

Move on to the next step if you have completed five ticks in a row. ✓

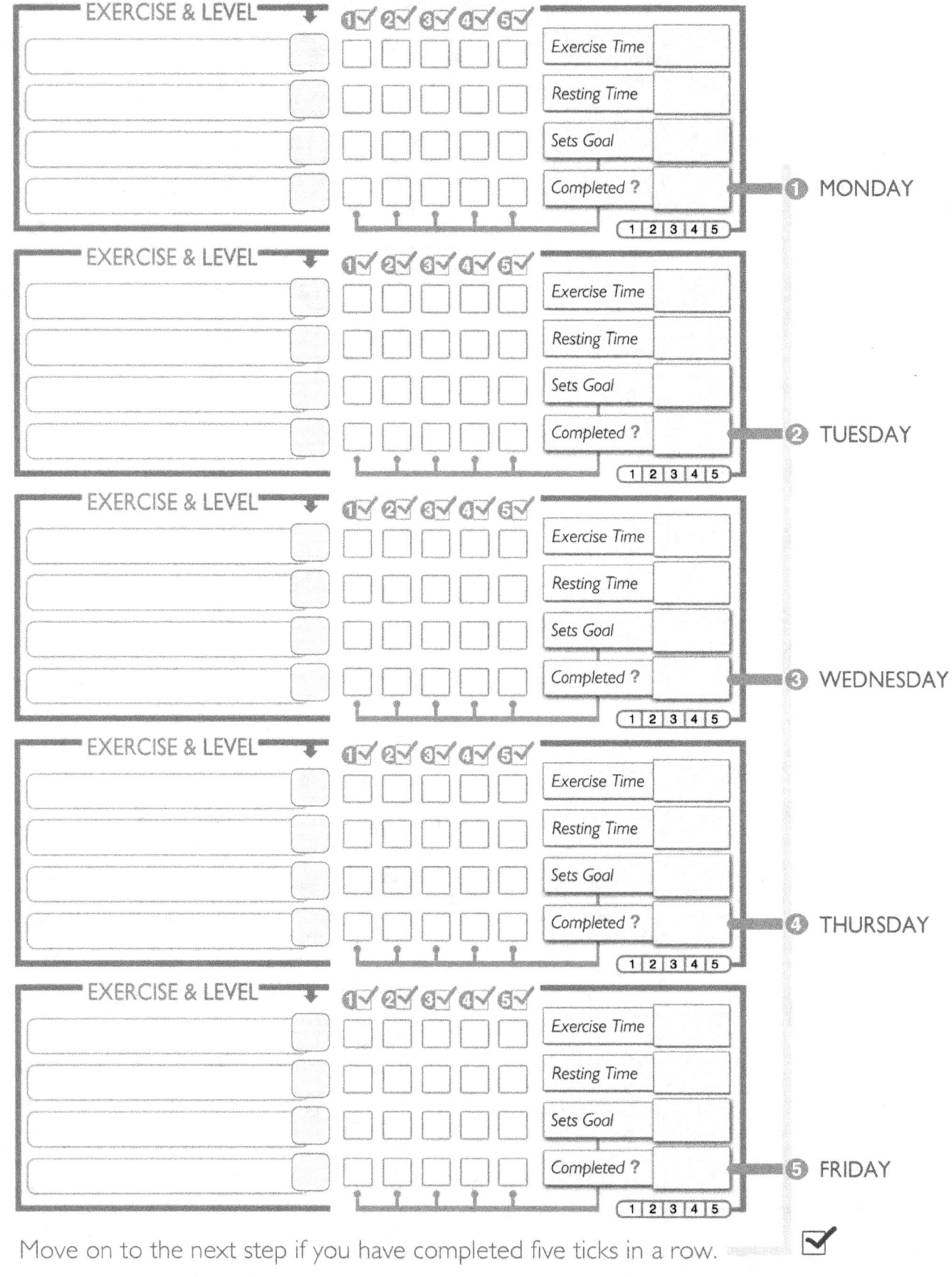

EXERCISE & LEVEL

1 2 3 4 5

Exercise Time

Resting Time

Sets Goal

Completed ?

1 MONDAY

1 2 3 4 5

EXERCISE & LEVEL

1 2 3 4 5

Exercise Time

Resting Time

Sets Goal

Completed ?

2 TUESDAY

1 2 3 4 5

EXERCISE & LEVEL

1 2 3 4 5

Exercise Time

Resting Time

Sets Goal

Completed ?

3 WEDNESDAY

1 2 3 4 5

EXERCISE & LEVEL

1 2 3 4 5

Exercise Time

Resting Time

Sets Goal

Completed ?

4 THURSDAY

1 2 3 4 5

EXERCISE & LEVEL

1 2 3 4 5

Exercise Time

Resting Time

Sets Goal

Completed ?

5 FRIDAY

1 2 3 4 5

Move on to the next step if you have completed five ticks in a row.

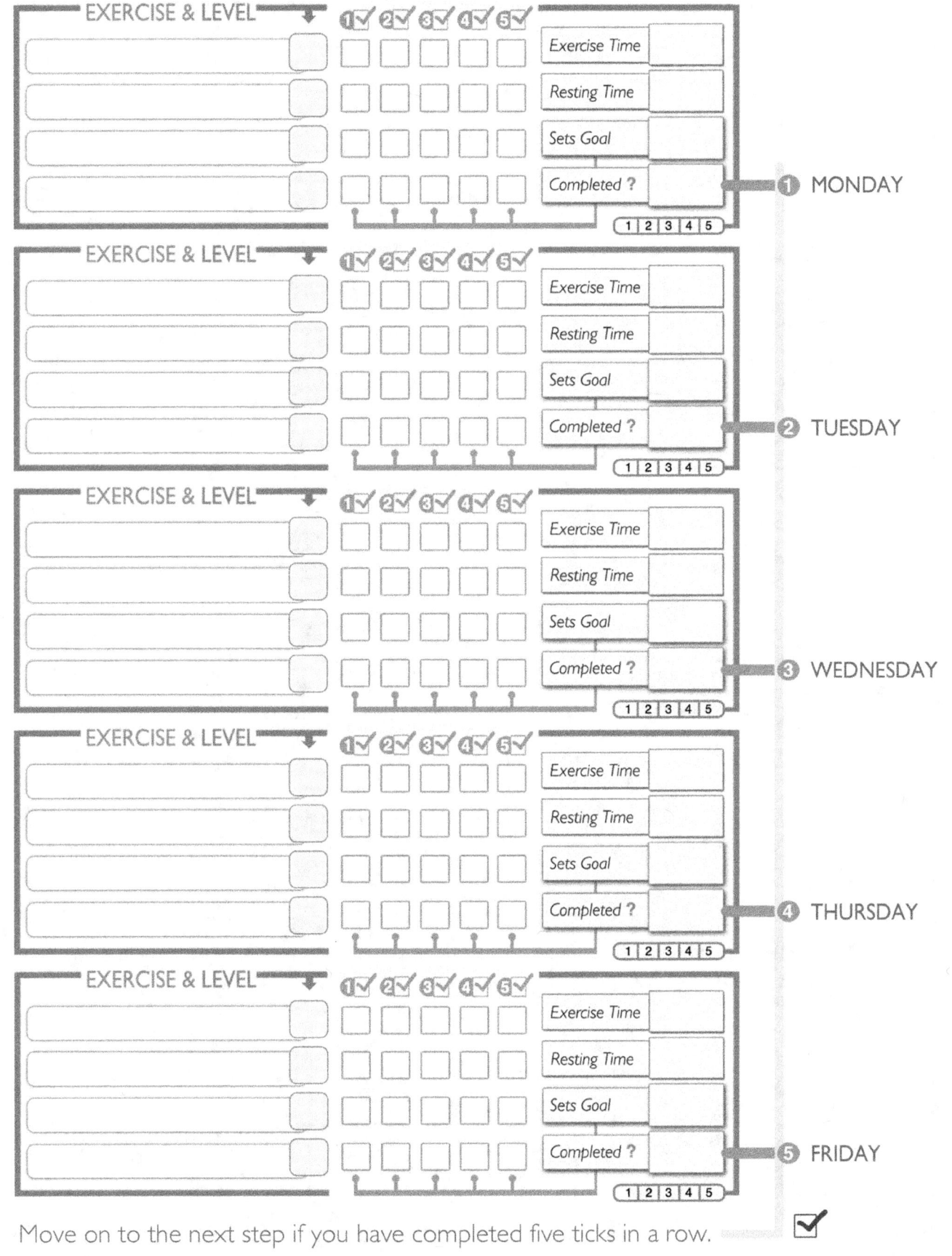

EXERCISE & LEVEL ①✓ ②✓ ③✓ ④✓ ⑤✓

Exercise Time
Resting Time
Sets Goal
Completed ?

1 2 3 4 5

1 MONDAY

EXERCISE & LEVEL ①✓ ②✓ ③✓ ④✓ ⑤✓

Exercise Time
Resting Time
Sets Goal
Completed ?

1 2 3 4 5

2 TUESDAY

EXERCISE & LEVEL ①✓ ②✓ ③✓ ④✓ ⑤✓

Exercise Time
Resting Time
Sets Goal
Completed ?

1 2 3 4 5

3 WEDNESDAY

EXERCISE & LEVEL ①✓ ②✓ ③✓ ④✓ ⑤✓

Exercise Time
Resting Time
Sets Goal
Completed ?

1 2 3 4 5

4 THURSDAY

EXERCISE & LEVEL ①✓ ②✓ ③✓ ④✓ ⑤✓

Exercise Time
Resting Time
Sets Goal
Completed ?

1 2 3 4 5

5 FRIDAY

Move on to the next step if you have completed five ticks in a row. ☑

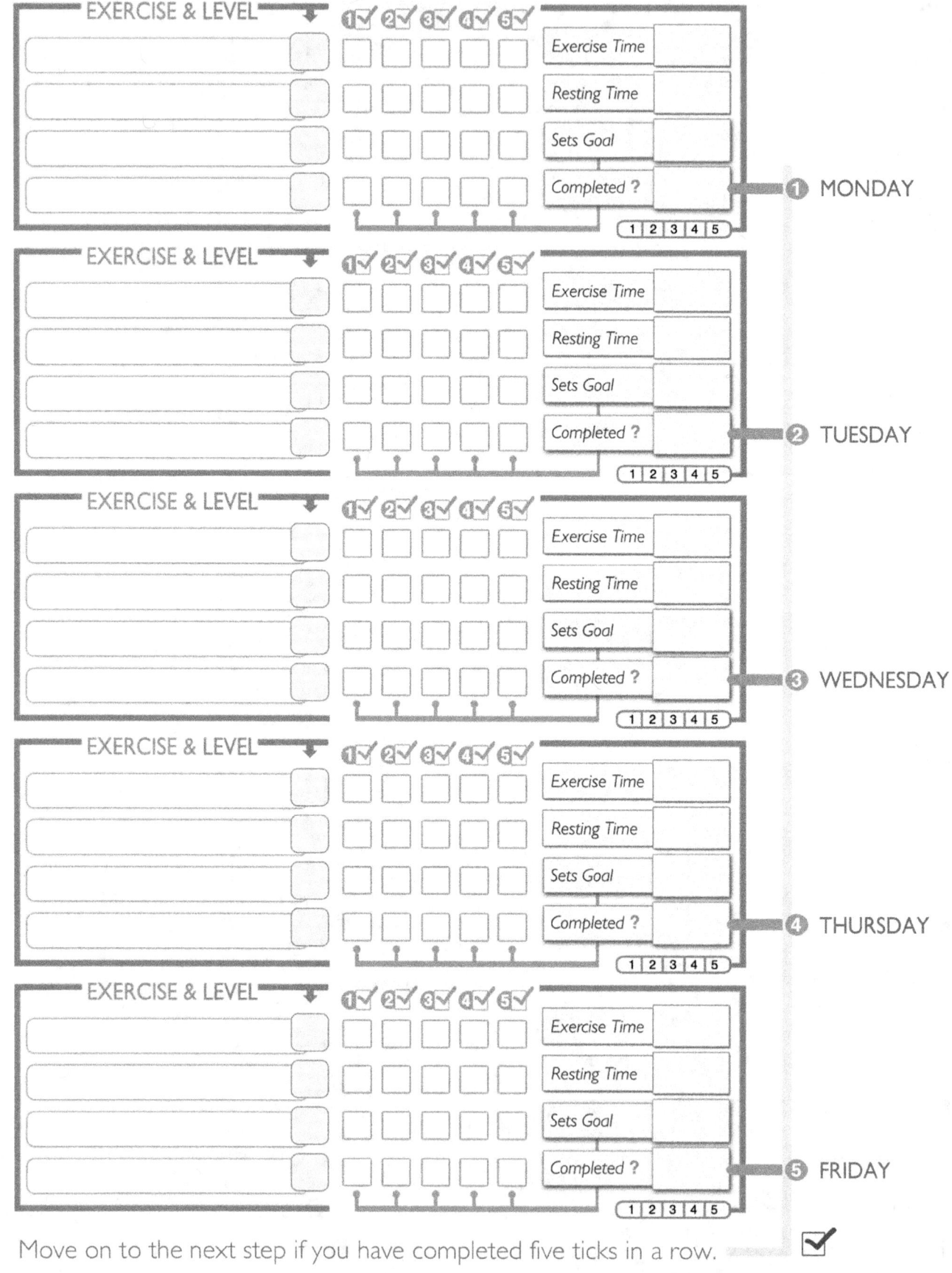

EXERCISE & LEVEL ▼ ①✓ ②✓ ③✓ ④✓ ⑤✓

Exercise Time
Resting Time
Sets Goal
Completed ?

1 2 3 4 5

1 MONDAY

EXERCISE & LEVEL ▼ ①✓ ②✓ ③✓ ④✓ ⑤✓

Exercise Time
Resting Time
Sets Goal
Completed ?

1 2 3 4 5

2 TUESDAY

EXERCISE & LEVEL ▼ ①✓ ②✓ ③✓ ④✓ ⑤✓

Exercise Time
Resting Time
Sets Goal
Completed ?

1 2 3 4 5

3 WEDNESDAY

EXERCISE & LEVEL ▼ ①✓ ②✓ ③✓ ④✓ ⑤✓

Exercise Time
Resting Time
Sets Goal
Completed ?

1 2 3 4 5

4 THURSDAY

EXERCISE & LEVEL ▼ ①✓ ②✓ ③✓ ④✓ ⑤✓

Exercise Time
Resting Time
Sets Goal
Completed ?

1 2 3 4 5

5 FRIDAY

Move on to the next step if you have completed five ticks in a row. ✓

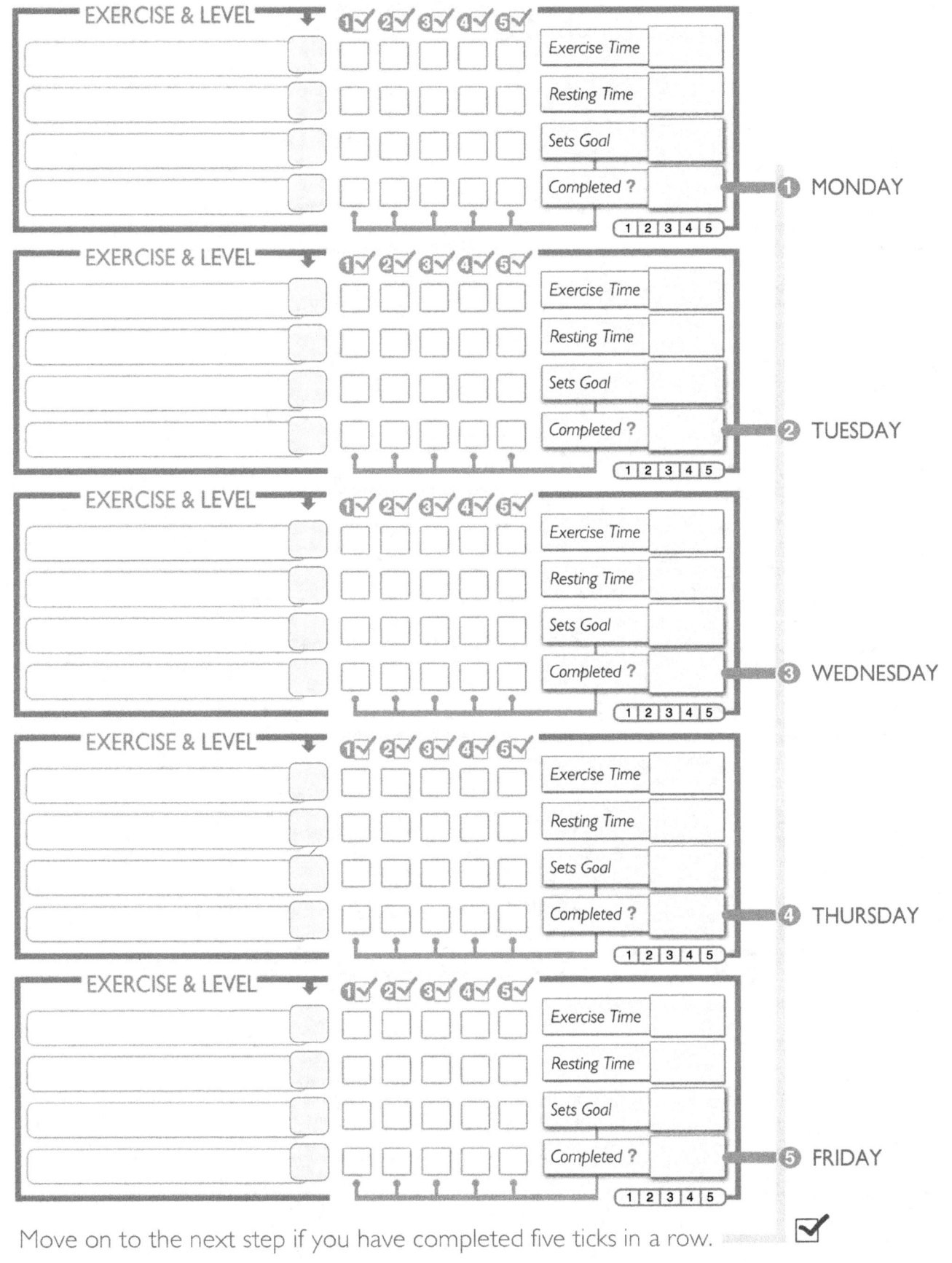

EXERCISE & LEVEL   1☑ 2☑ 3☑ 4☑ 5☑   Exercise Time / Resting Time / Sets Goal / Completed ?   1 2 3 4 5   **1 MONDAY**

EXERCISE & LEVEL   1☑ 2☑ 3☑ 4☑ 5☑   Exercise Time / Resting Time / Sets Goal / Completed ?   1 2 3 4 5   **2 TUESDAY**

EXERCISE & LEVEL   1☑ 2☑ 3☑ 4☑ 5☑   Exercise Time / Resting Time / Sets Goal / Completed ?   1 2 3 4 5   **3 WEDNESDAY**

EXERCISE & LEVEL   1☑ 2☑ 3☑ 4☑ 5☑   Exercise Time / Resting Time / Sets Goal / Completed ?   1 2 3 4 5   **4 THURSDAY**

EXERCISE & LEVEL   1☑ 2☑ 3☑ 4☑ 5☑   Exercise Time / Resting Time / Sets Goal / Completed ?   1 2 3 4 5   **5 FRIDAY**

Move on to the next step if you have completed five ticks in a row. ☑

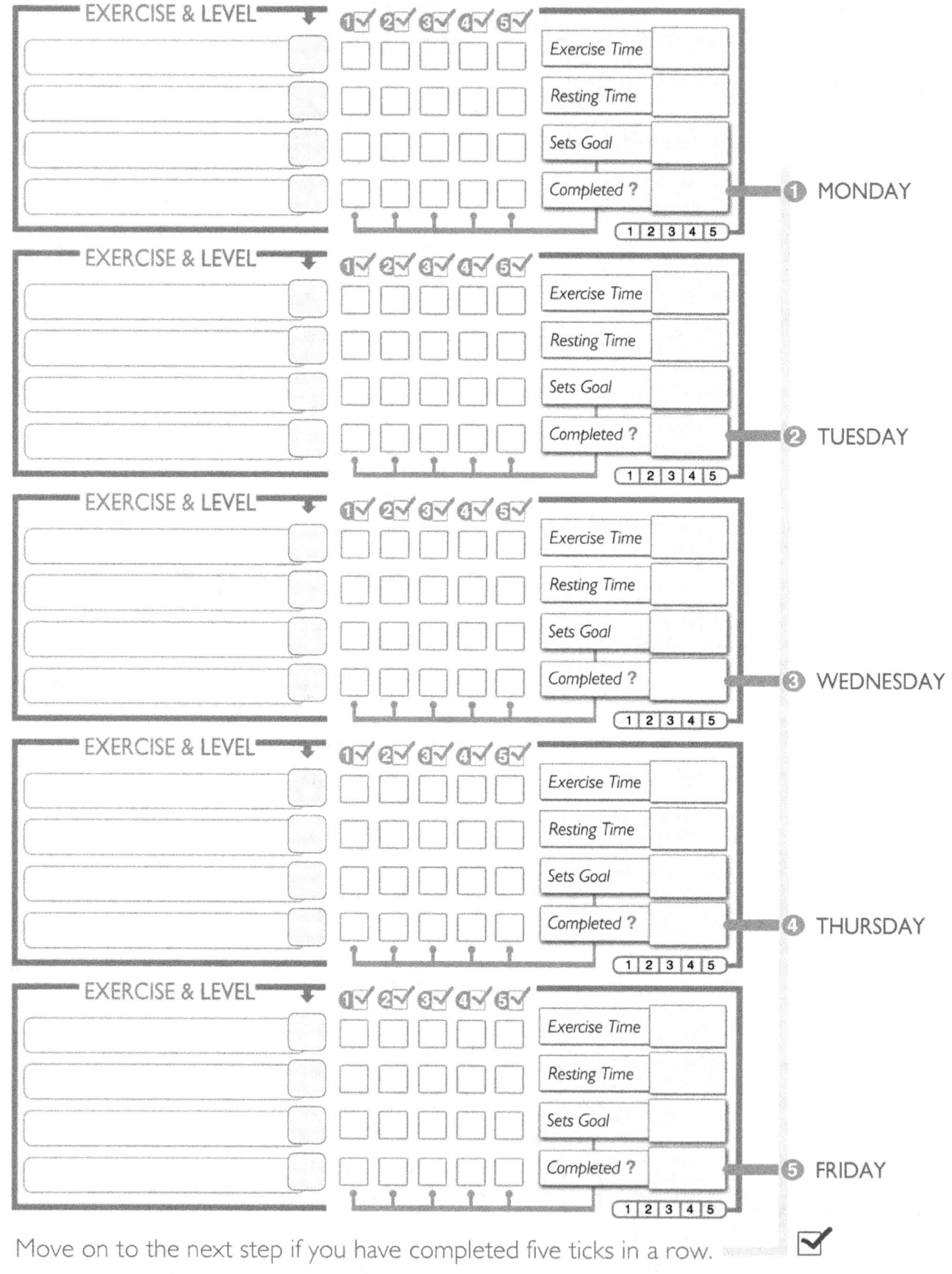

EXERCISE & LEVEL 1✓ 2✓ 3✓ 4✓ 5✓

Exercise Time
Resting Time
Sets Goal
Completed ?

1 MONDAY

1 2 3 4 5

EXERCISE & LEVEL 1✓ 2✓ 3✓ 4✓ 5✓

Exercise Time
Resting Time
Sets Goal
Completed ?

2 TUESDAY

1 2 3 4 5

EXERCISE & LEVEL 1✓ 2✓ 3✓ 4✓ 5✓

Exercise Time
Resting Time
Sets Goal
Completed ?

3 WEDNESDAY

1 2 3 4 5

EXERCISE & LEVEL 1✓ 2✓ 3✓ 4✓ 5✓

Exercise Time
Resting Time
Sets Goal
Completed ?

4 THURSDAY

1 2 3 4 5

EXERCISE & LEVEL 1✓ 2✓ 3✓ 4✓ 5✓

Exercise Time
Resting Time
Sets Goal
Completed ?

5 FRIDAY

1 2 3 4 5

Move on to the next step if you have completed five ticks in a row. ✓

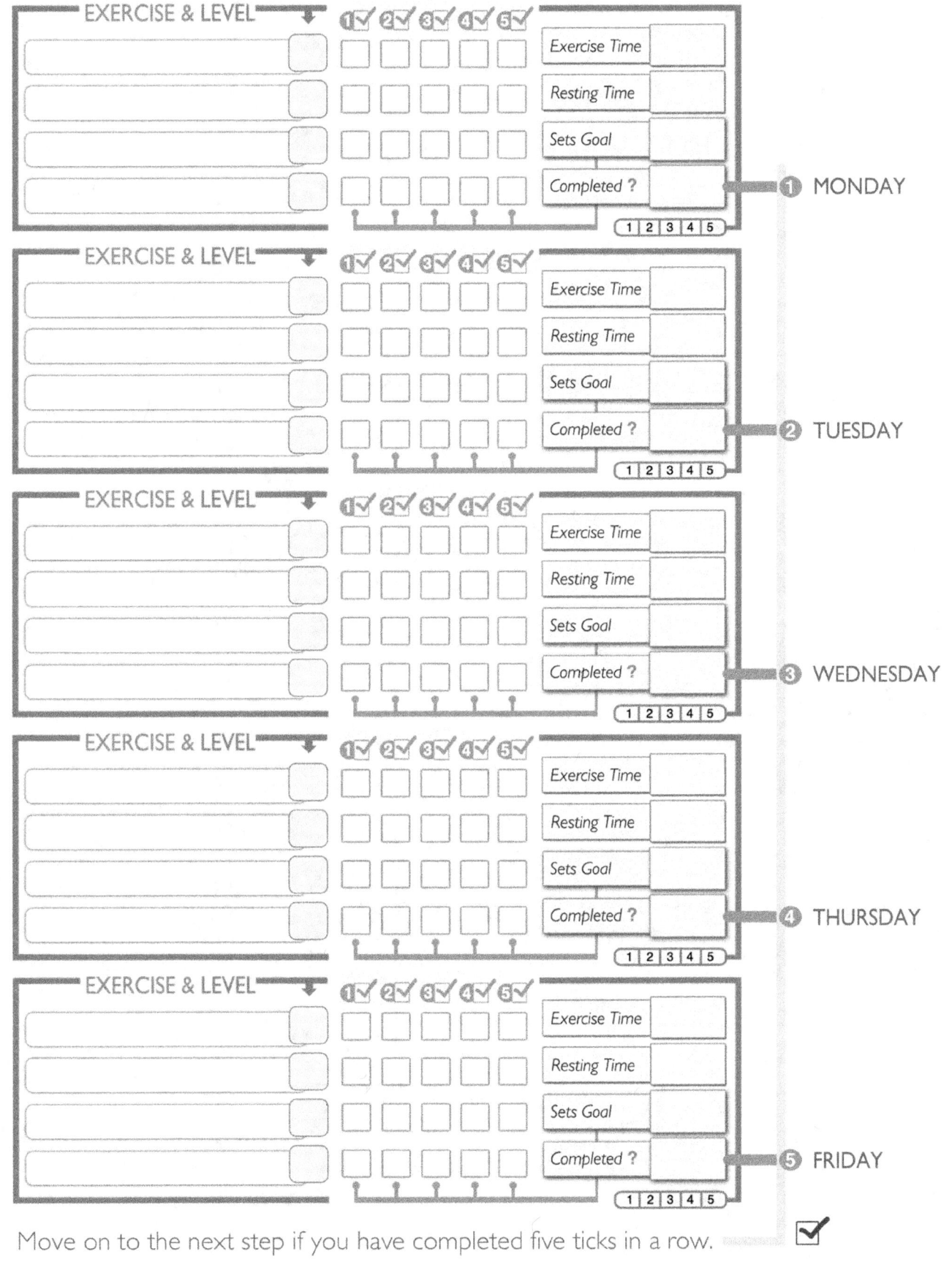

EXERCISE & LEVEL   ① ② ③ ④ ⑤

Exercise Time
Resting Time
Sets Goal
Completed ?   ① MONDAY
1 2 3 4 5

EXERCISE & LEVEL   ① ② ③ ④ ⑤

Exercise Time
Resting Time
Sets Goal
Completed ?   ② TUESDAY
1 2 3 4 5

EXERCISE & LEVEL   ① ② ③ ④ ⑤

Exercise Time
Resting Time
Sets Goal
Completed ?   ③ WEDNESDAY
1 2 3 4 5

EXERCISE & LEVEL   ① ② ③ ④ ⑤

Exercise Time
Resting Time
Sets Goal
Completed ?   ④ THURSDAY
1 2 3 4 5

EXERCISE & LEVEL   ① ② ③ ④ ⑤

Exercise Time
Resting Time
Sets Goal
Completed ?   ⑤ FRIDAY
1 2 3 4 5

Move on to the next step if you have completed five ticks in a row. ✔

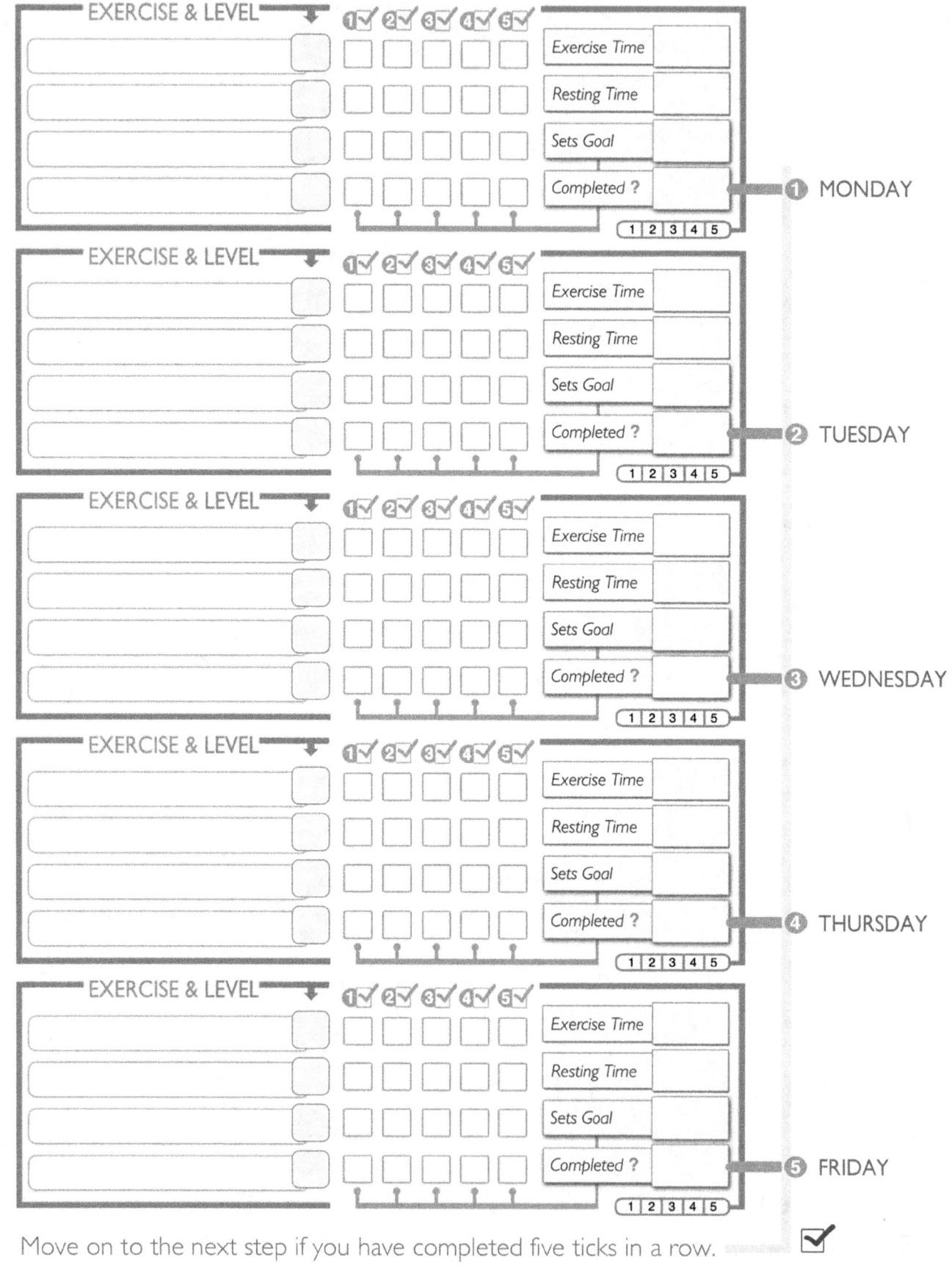

Move on to the next step if you have completed five ticks in a row.

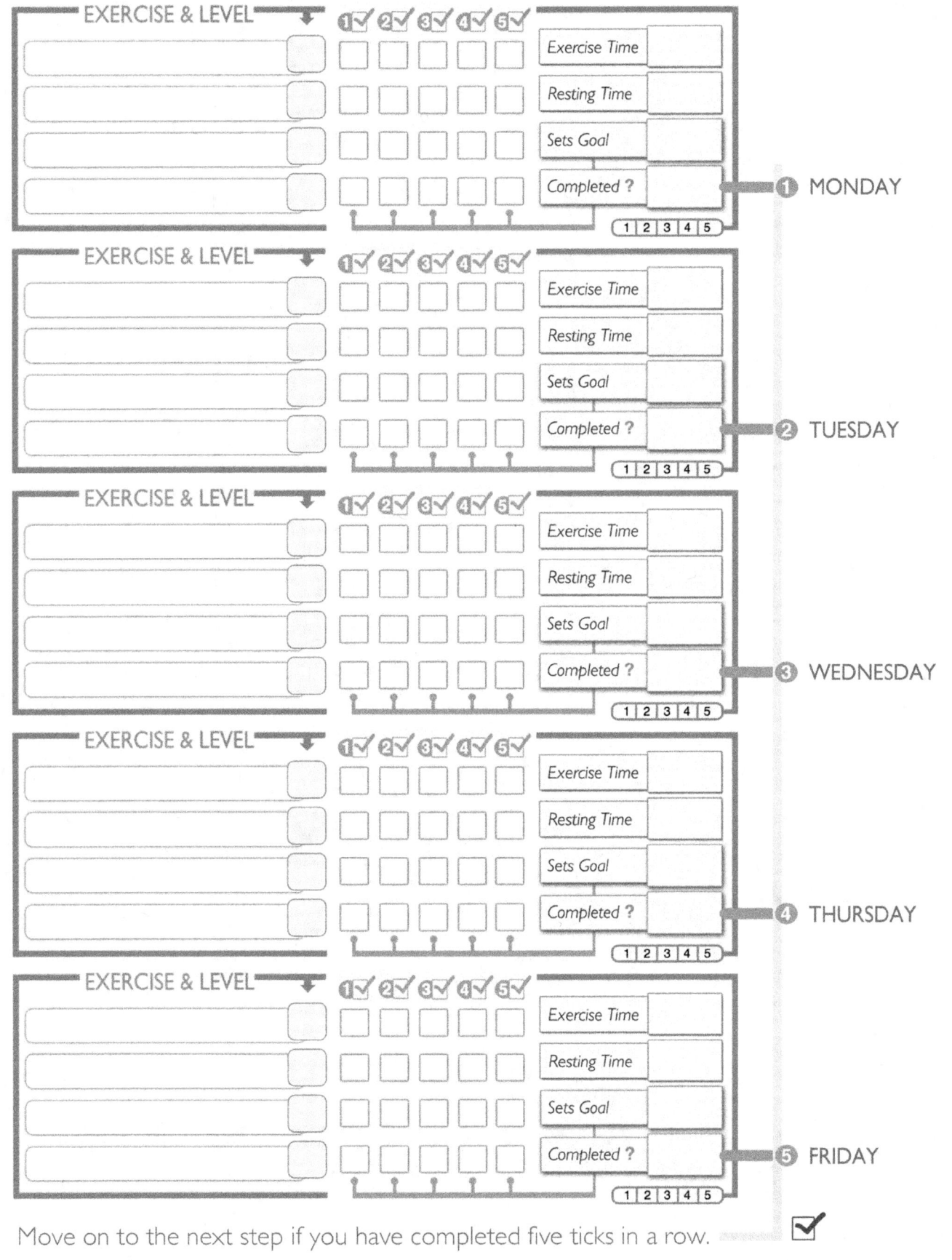

EXERCISE & LEVEL

1 2 3 4 5

Exercise Time	
Resting Time	
Sets Goal	
Completed ?	

1 2 3 4 5

1 MONDAY

EXERCISE & LEVEL

1 2 3 4 5

Exercise Time	
Resting Time	
Sets Goal	
Completed ?	

1 2 3 4 5

2 TUESDAY

EXERCISE & LEVEL

1 2 3 4 5

Exercise Time	
Resting Time	
Sets Goal	
Completed ?	

1 2 3 4 5

3 WEDNESDAY

EXERCISE & LEVEL

1 2 3 4 5

Exercise Time	
Resting Time	
Sets Goal	
Completed ?	

1 2 3 4 5

4 THURSDAY

EXERCISE & LEVEL

1 2 3 4 5

Exercise Time	
Resting Time	
Sets Goal	
Completed ?	

1 2 3 4 5

5 FRIDAY

Move on to the next step if you have completed five ticks in a row.

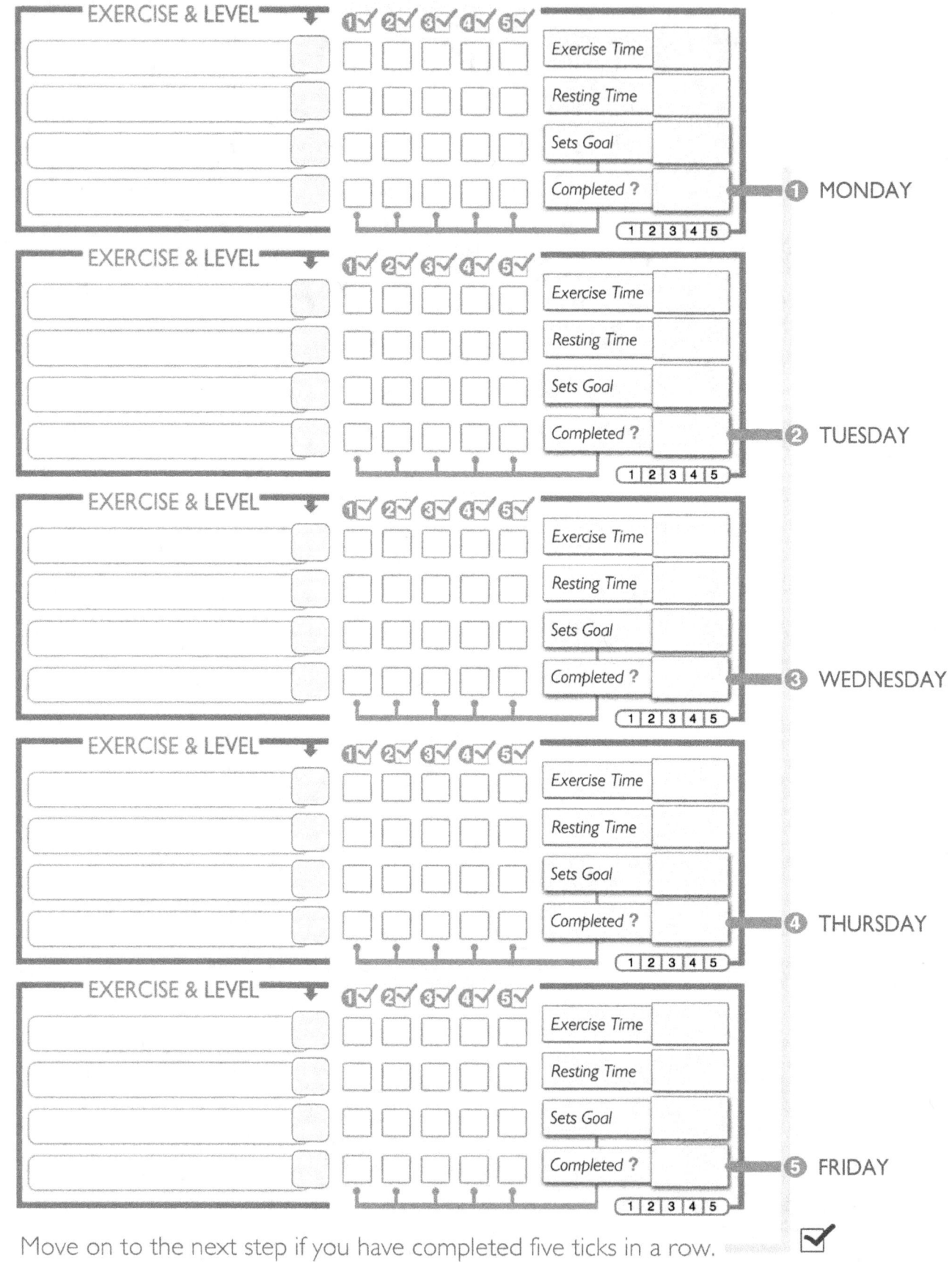

EXERCISE & LEVEL

1 2 3 4 5

Exercise Time
Resting Time
Sets Goal
Completed ?

1 2 3 4 5

1 MONDAY

EXERCISE & LEVEL

1 2 3 4 5

Exercise Time
Resting Time
Sets Goal
Completed ?

1 2 3 4 5

2 TUESDAY

EXERCISE & LEVEL

1 2 3 4 5

Exercise Time
Resting Time
Sets Goal
Completed ?

1 2 3 4 5

3 WEDNESDAY

EXERCISE & LEVEL

1 2 3 4 5

Exercise Time
Resting Time
Sets Goal
Completed ?

1 2 3 4 5

4 THURSDAY

EXERCISE & LEVEL

1 2 3 4 5

Exercise Time
Resting Time
Sets Goal
Completed ?

1 2 3 4 5

5 FRIDAY

Move on to the next step if you have completed five ticks in a row.

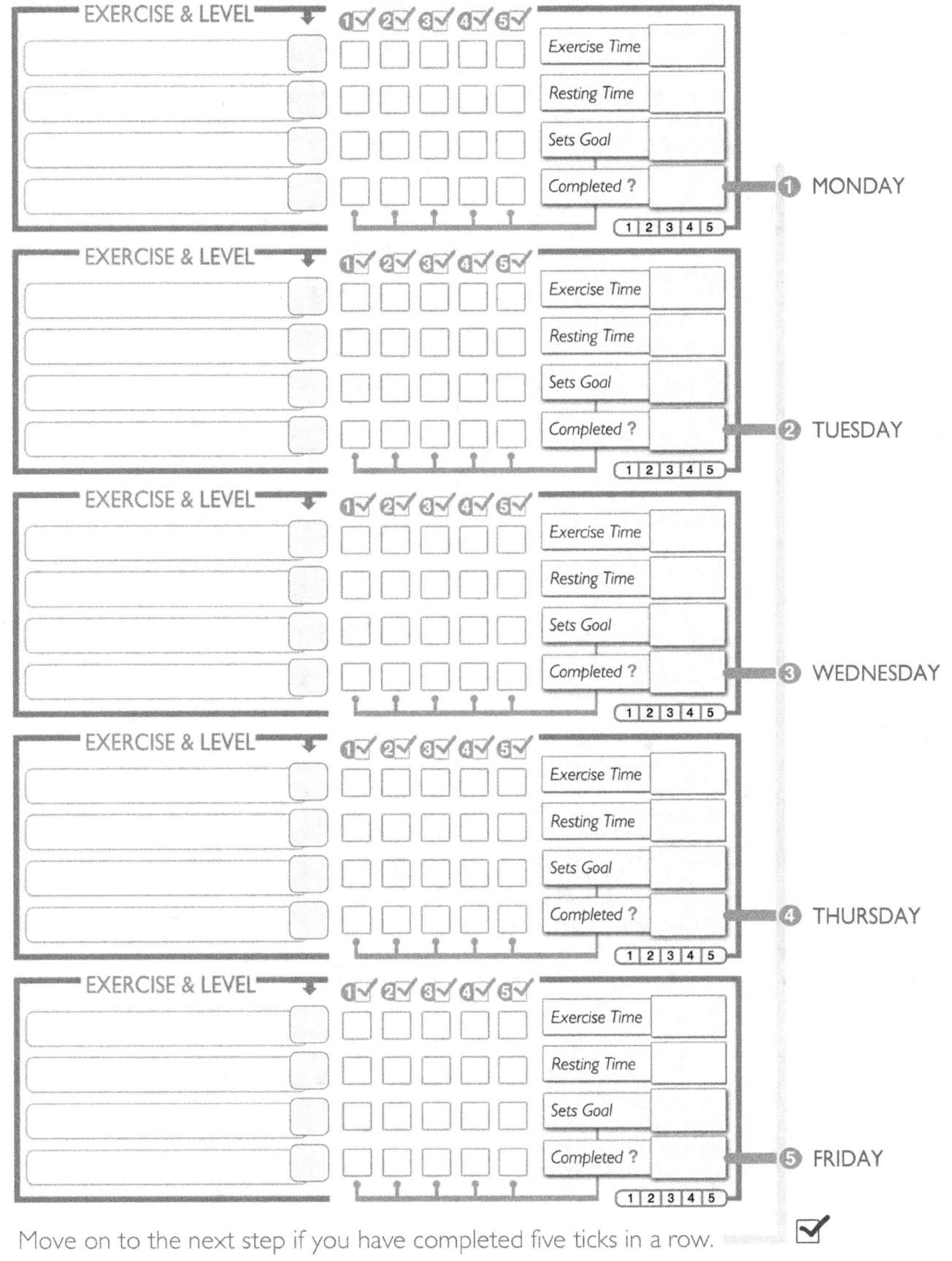

EXERCISE & LEVEL | 1✓ 2✓ 3✓ 4✓ 5✓

Exercise Time
Resting Time
Sets Goal
Completed ?

❶ MONDAY

1 2 3 4 5

EXERCISE & LEVEL | 1✓ 2✓ 3✓ 4✓ 5✓

Exercise Time
Resting Time
Sets Goal
Completed ?

❷ TUESDAY

1 2 3 4 5

EXERCISE & LEVEL | 1✓ 2✓ 3✓ 4✓ 5✓

Exercise Time
Resting Time
Sets Goal
Completed ?

❸ WEDNESDAY

1 2 3 4 5

EXERCISE & LEVEL | 1✓ 2✓ 3✓ 4✓ 5✓

Exercise Time
Resting Time
Sets Goal
Completed ?

❹ THURSDAY

1 2 3 4 5

EXERCISE & LEVEL | 1✓ 2✓ 3✓ 4✓ 5✓

Exercise Time
Resting Time
Sets Goal
Completed ?

❺ FRIDAY

1 2 3 4 5

Move on to the next step if you have completed five ticks in a row. ✓

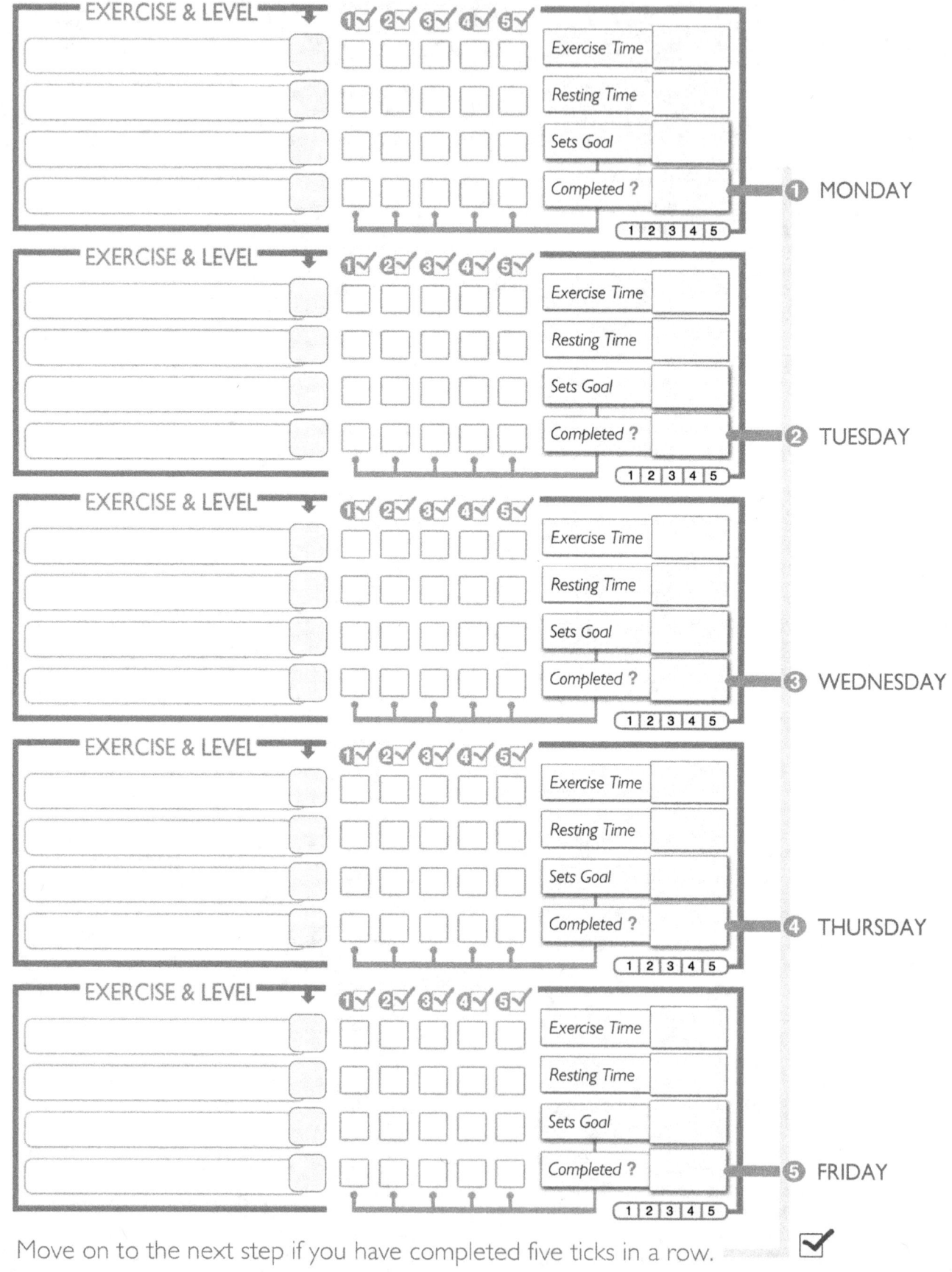

EXERCISE & LEVEL

Exercise Time
Resting Time
Sets Goal
Completed ?

1 MONDAY

2 TUESDAY

3 WEDNESDAY

4 THURSDAY

5 FRIDAY

Move on to the next step if you have completed five ticks in a row.

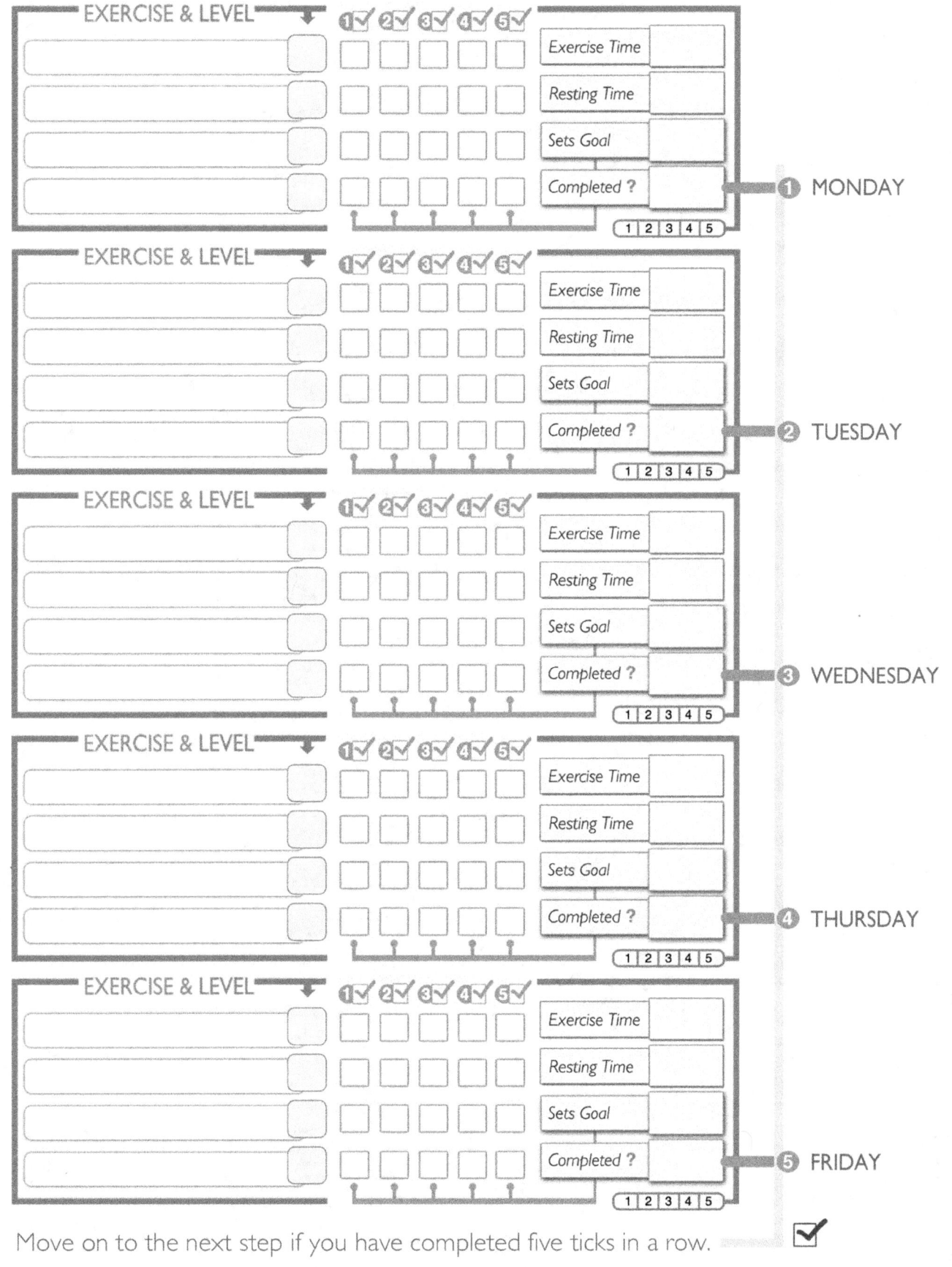

Move on to the next step if you have completed five ticks in a row. ☑

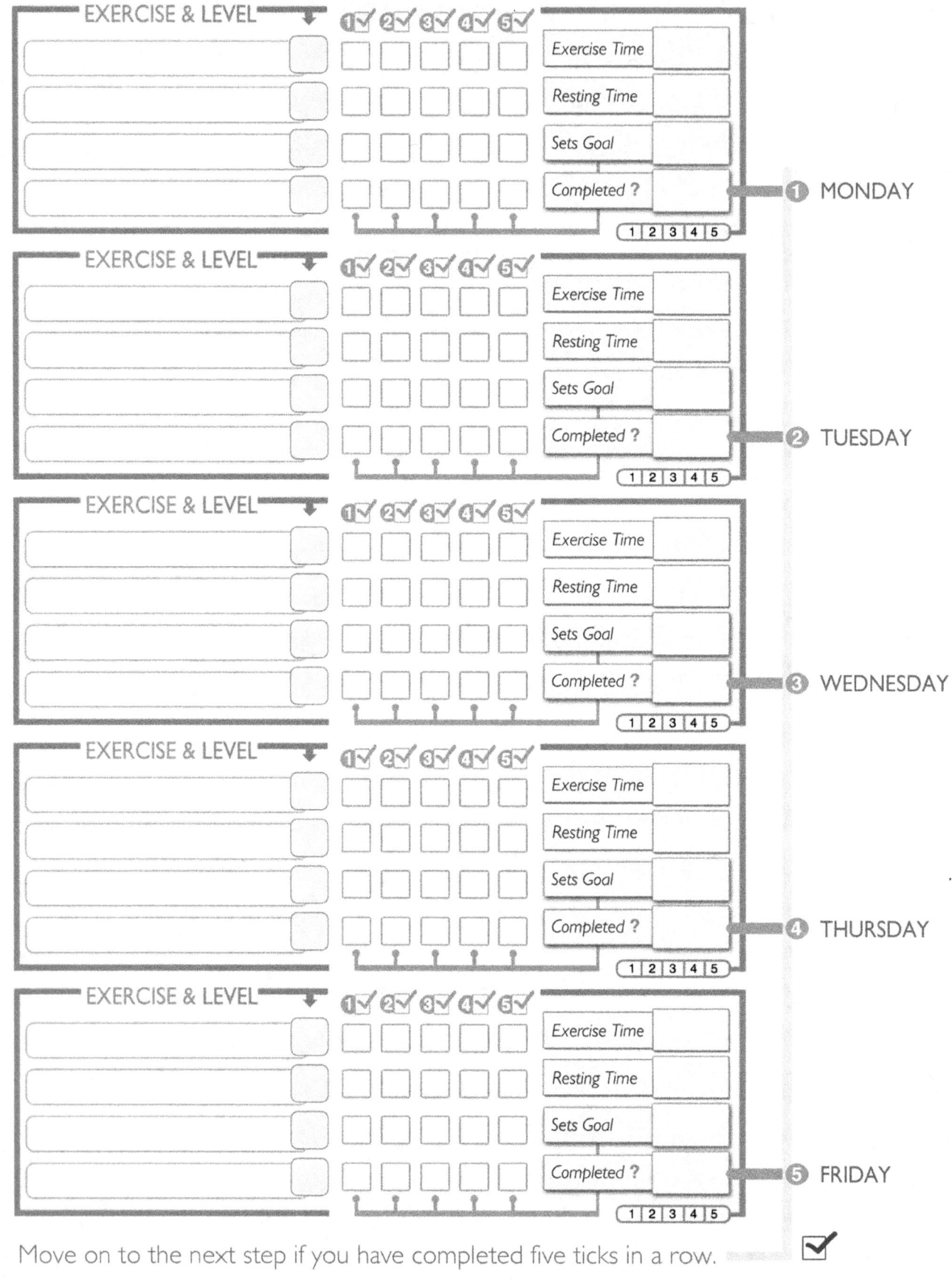

EXERCISE & LEVEL · 1✓ 2✓ 3✓ 4✓ 5✓ · Exercise Time · Resting Time · Sets Goal · Completed ? · 1 2 3 4 5 · ❶ MONDAY

EXERCISE & LEVEL · 1✓ 2✓ 3✓ 4✓ 5✓ · Exercise Time · Resting Time · Sets Goal · Completed ? · 1 2 3 4 5 · ❷ TUESDAY

EXERCISE & LEVEL · 1✓ 2✓ 3✓ 4✓ 5✓ · Exercise Time · Resting Time · Sets Goal · Completed ? · 1 2 3 4 5 · ❸ WEDNESDAY

EXERCISE & LEVEL · 1✓ 2✓ 3✓ 4✓ 5✓ · Exercise Time · Resting Time · Sets Goal · Completed ? · 1 2 3 4 5 · ❹ THURSDAY

EXERCISE & LEVEL · 1✓ 2✓ 3✓ 4✓ 5✓ · Exercise Time · Resting Time · Sets Goal · Completed ? · 1 2 3 4 5 · ❺ FRIDAY

Move on to the next step if you have completed five ticks in a row. ☑

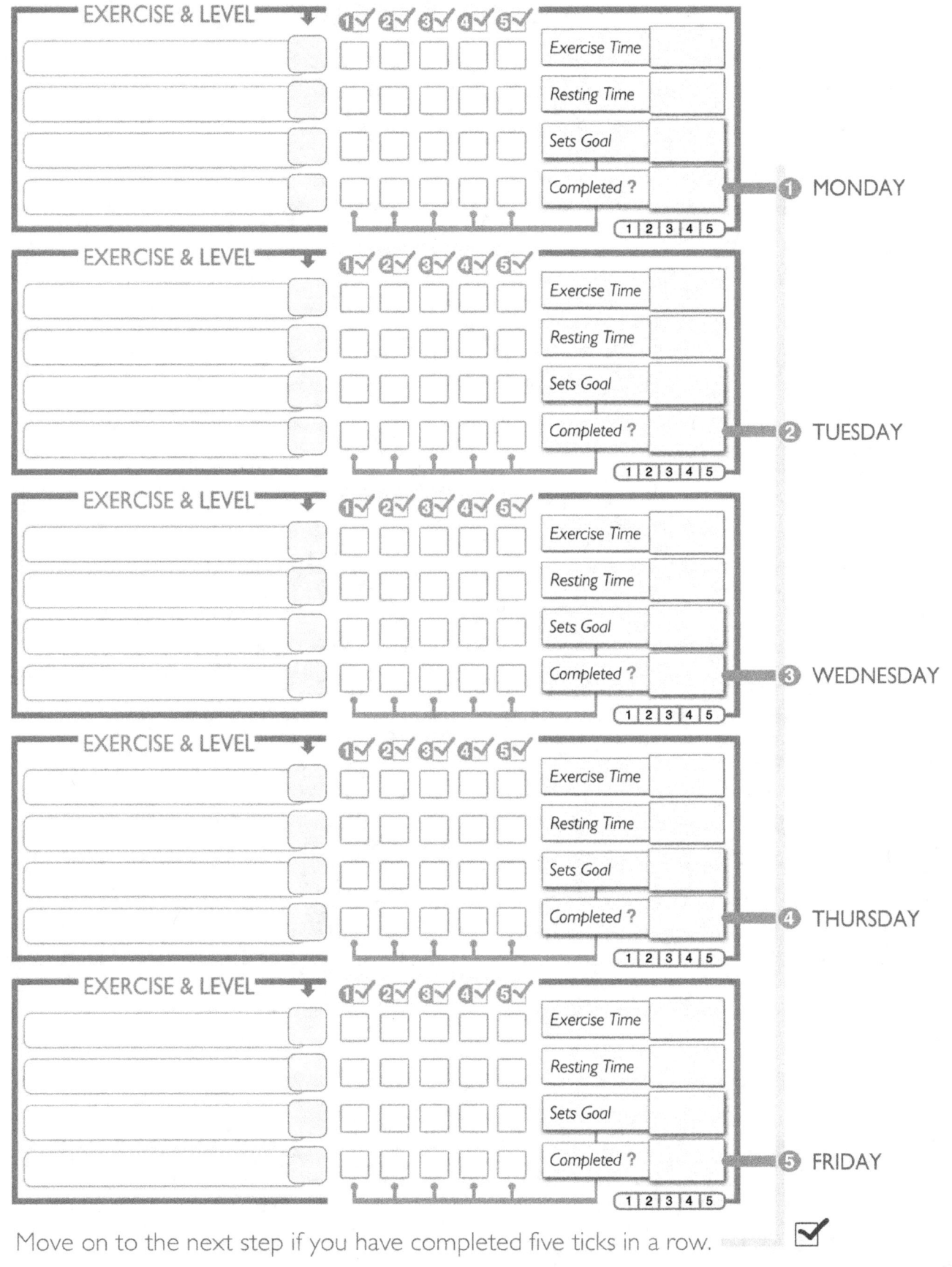

EXERCISE & LEVEL

1 ✓ 2 ✓ 3 ✓ 4 ✓ 5 ✓

Exercise Time
Resting Time
Sets Goal
Completed ?

1 | 2 | 3 | 4 | 5

1 MONDAY

EXERCISE & LEVEL

1 ✓ 2 ✓ 3 ✓ 4 ✓ 5 ✓

Exercise Time
Resting Time
Sets Goal
Completed ?

1 | 2 | 3 | 4 | 5

2 TUESDAY

EXERCISE & LEVEL

1 ✓ 2 ✓ 3 ✓ 4 ✓ 5 ✓

Exercise Time
Resting Time
Sets Goal
Completed ?

1 | 2 | 3 | 4 | 5

3 WEDNESDAY

EXERCISE & LEVEL

1 ✓ 2 ✓ 3 ✓ 4 ✓ 5 ✓

Exercise Time
Resting Time
Sets Goal
Completed ?

1 | 2 | 3 | 4 | 5

4 THURSDAY

EXERCISE & LEVEL

1 ✓ 2 ✓ 3 ✓ 4 ✓ 5 ✓

Exercise Time
Resting Time
Sets Goal
Completed ?

1 | 2 | 3 | 4 | 5

5 FRIDAY

Move on to the next step if you have completed five ticks in a row. ✓

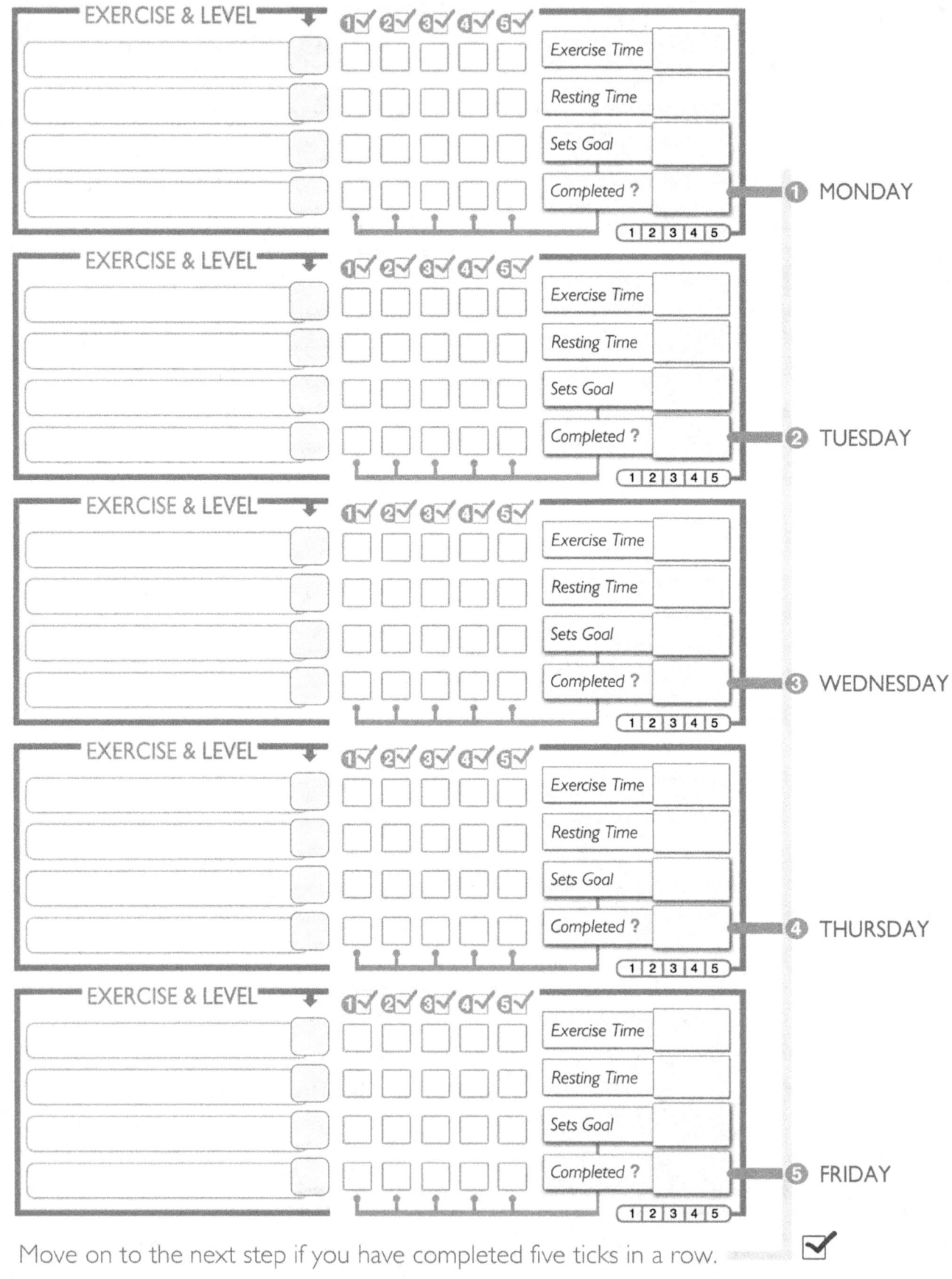

Move on to the next step if you have completed five ticks in a row.

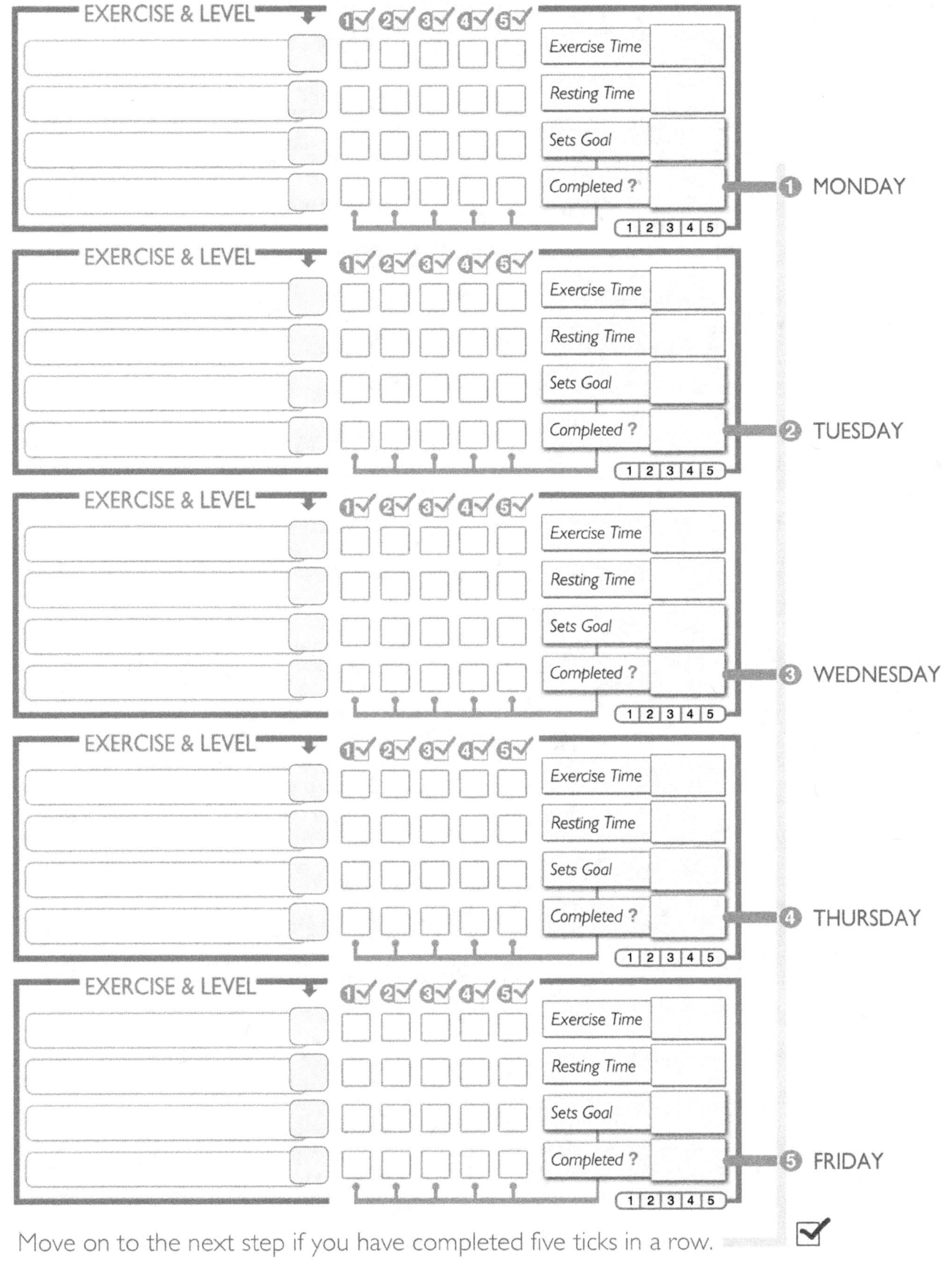

EXERCISE & LEVEL

1☑ 2☑ 3☑ 4☑ 5☑

Exercise Time

Resting Time

Sets Goal

Completed ?

1 2 3 4 5

1 MONDAY

EXERCISE & LEVEL

1☑ 2☑ 3☑ 4☑ 5☑

Exercise Time

Resting Time

Sets Goal

Completed ?

1 2 3 4 5

2 TUESDAY

EXERCISE & LEVEL

1☑ 2☑ 3☑ 4☑ 5☑

Exercise Time

Resting Time

Sets Goal

Completed ?

1 2 3 4 5

3 WEDNESDAY

EXERCISE & LEVEL

1☑ 2☑ 3☑ 4☑ 5☑

Exercise Time

Resting Time

Sets Goal

Completed ?

1 2 3 4 5

4 THURSDAY

EXERCISE & LEVEL

1☑ 2☑ 3☑ 4☑ 5☑

Exercise Time

Resting Time

Sets Goal

Completed ?

1 2 3 4 5

5 FRIDAY

Move on to the next step if you have completed five ticks in a row. ☑

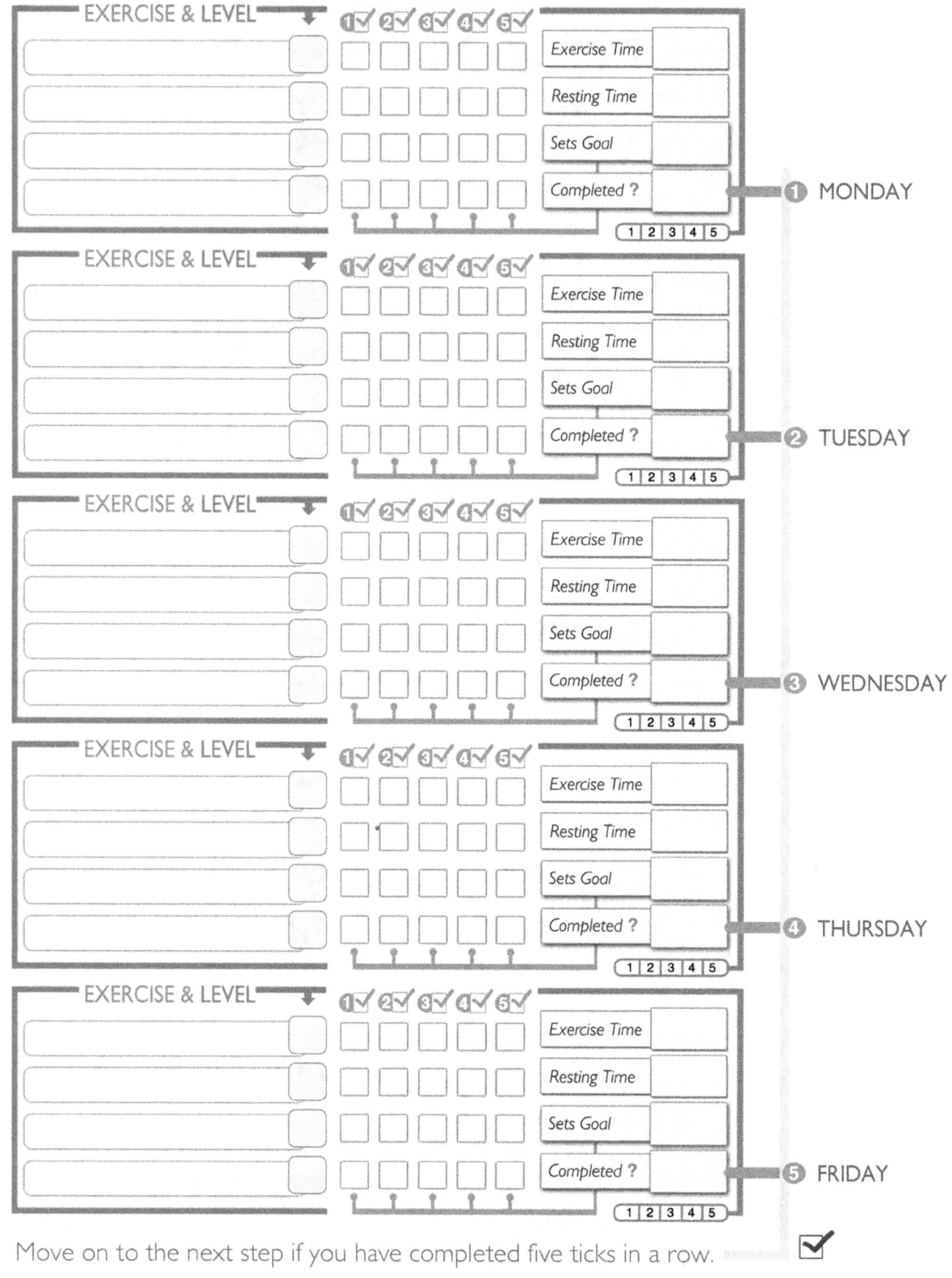

| | | | | | EXERCISE & LEVEL | 1 ✓ | 2 ✓ | 3 ✓ | 4 ✓ | 5 ✓ |

① MONDAY

Exercise Time
Resting Time
Sets Goal
Completed ?

1 2 3 4 5

② TUESDAY

Exercise Time
Resting Time
Sets Goal
Completed ?

1 2 3 4 5

③ WEDNESDAY

Exercise Time
Resting Time
Sets Goal
Completed ?

1 2 3 4 5

④ THURSDAY

Exercise Time
Resting Time
Sets Goal
Completed ?

1 2 3 4 5

⑤ FRIDAY

Exercise Time
Resting Time
Sets Goal
Completed ?

1 2 3 4 5

Move on to the next step if you have completed five ticks in a row. ☑

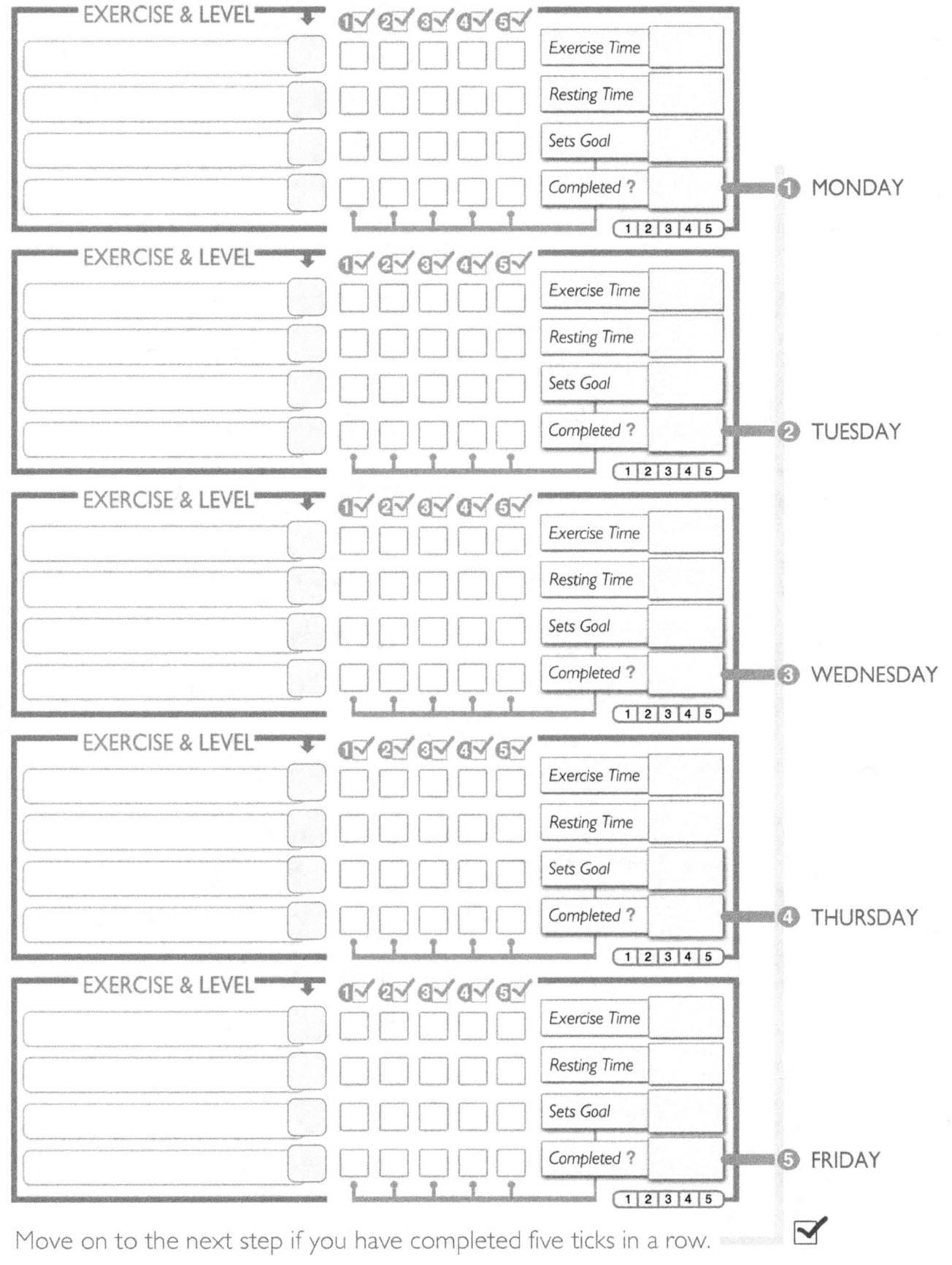

EXERCISE & LEVEL | 1✓ 2✓ 3✓ 4✓ 5✓

Exercise Time
Resting Time
Sets Goal
Completed ?

1 2 3 4 5

1 MONDAY

EXERCISE & LEVEL | 1✓ 2✓ 3✓ 4✓ 5✓

Exercise Time
Resting Time
Sets Goal
Completed ?

1 2 3 4 5

2 TUESDAY

EXERCISE & LEVEL | 1✓ 2✓ 3✓ 4✓ 5✓

Exercise Time
Resting Time
Sets Goal
Completed ?

1 2 3 4 5

3 WEDNESDAY

EXERCISE & LEVEL | 1✓ 2✓ 3✓ 4✓ 5✓

Exercise Time
Resting Time
Sets Goal
Completed ?

1 2 3 4 5

4 THURSDAY

EXERCISE & LEVEL | 1✓ 2✓ 3✓ 4✓ 5✓

Exercise Time
Resting Time
Sets Goal
Completed ?

1 2 3 4 5

5 FRIDAY

Move on to the next step if you have completed five ticks in a row. ✓

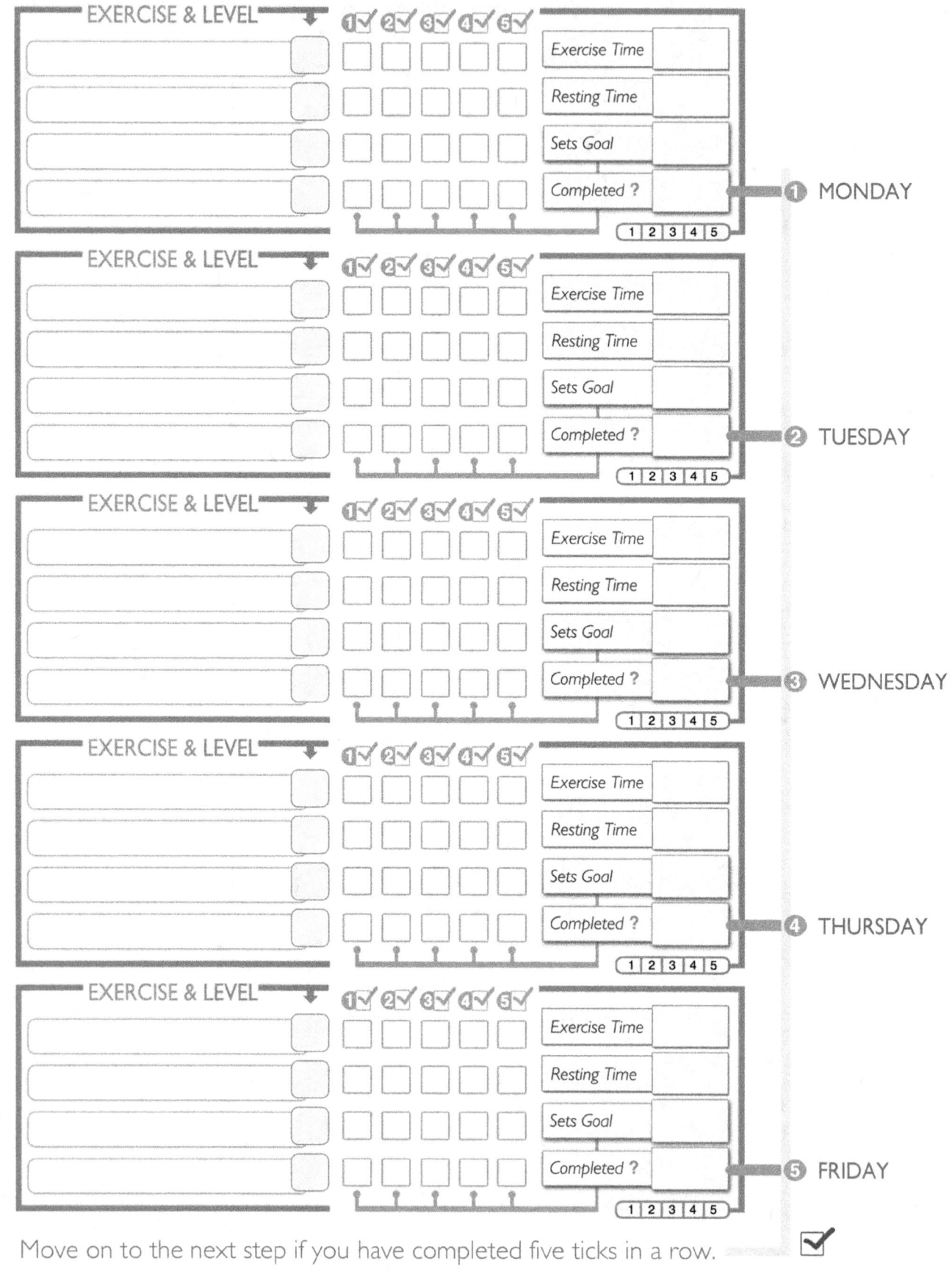

EXERCISE & LEVEL ① ✓ ② ✓ ③ ✓ ④ ✓ ⑤ ✓

Exercise Time
Resting Time
Sets Goal
Completed ?
❶ MONDAY
1 2 3 4 5

EXERCISE & LEVEL ① ✓ ② ✓ ③ ✓ ④ ✓ ⑤ ✓

Exercise Time
Resting Time
Sets Goal
Completed ?
❷ TUESDAY
1 2 3 4 5

EXERCISE & LEVEL ① ✓ ② ✓ ③ ✓ ④ ✓ ⑤ ✓

Exercise Time
Resting Time
Sets Goal
Completed ?
❸ WEDNESDAY
1 2 3 4 5

EXERCISE & LEVEL ① ✓ ② ✓ ③ ✓ ④ ✓ ⑤ ✓

Exercise Time
Resting Time
Sets Goal
Completed ?
❹ THURSDAY
1 2 3 4 5

EXERCISE & LEVEL ① ✓ ② ✓ ③ ✓ ④ ✓ ⑤ ✓

Exercise Time
Resting Time
Sets Goal
Completed ?
❺ FRIDAY
1 2 3 4 5

Move on to the next step if you have completed five ticks in a row. ✓

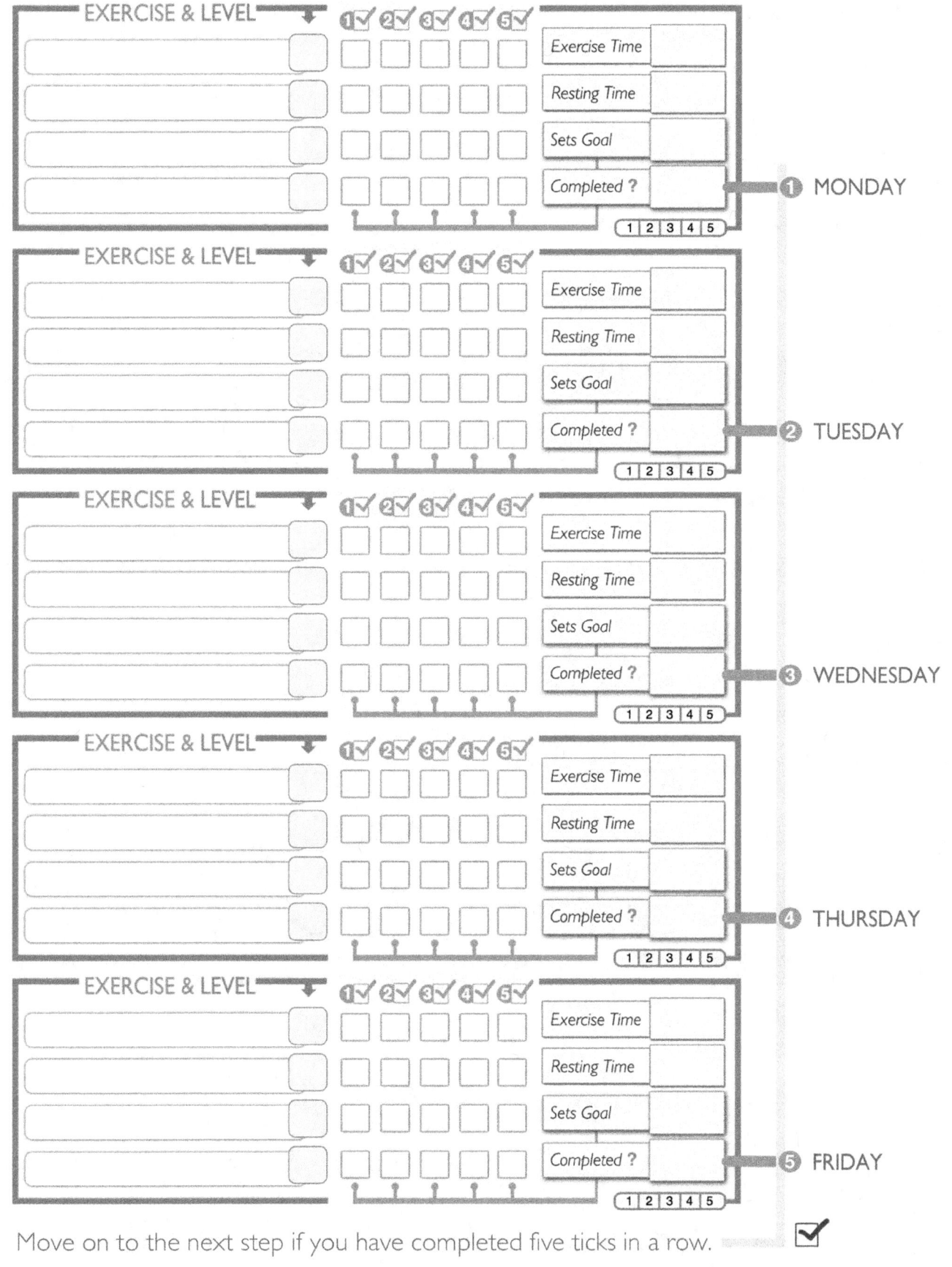

EXERCISE & LEVEL

① ② ③ ④ ⑤

Exercise Time

Resting Time

Sets Goal

Completed ?

1 2 3 4 5

① MONDAY

② TUESDAY

③ WEDNESDAY

④ THURSDAY

⑤ FRIDAY

Move on to the next step if you have completed five ticks in a row.

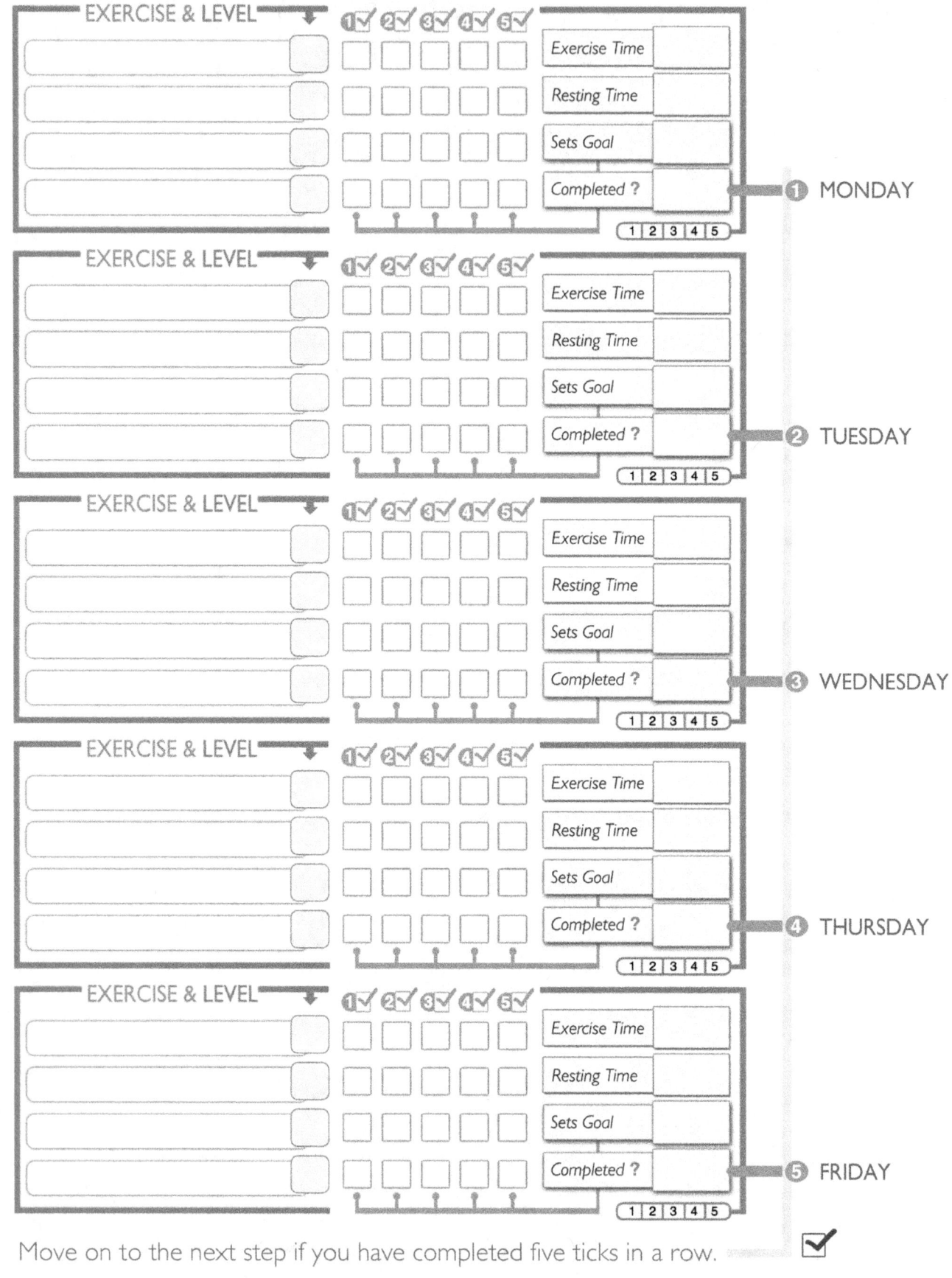

EXERCISE & LEVEL   ① ② ③ ④ ⑤

Exercise Time	
Resting Time	
Sets Goal	
Completed ?	

❶ MONDAY

1 2 3 4 5

EXERCISE & LEVEL   ① ② ③ ④ ⑤

Exercise Time	
Resting Time	
Sets Goal	
Completed ?	

❷ TUESDAY

1 2 3 4 5

EXERCISE & LEVEL   ① ② ③ ④ ⑤

Exercise Time	
Resting Time	
Sets Goal	
Completed ?	

❸ WEDNESDAY

1 2 3 4 5

EXERCISE & LEVEL   ① ② ③ ④ ⑤

Exercise Time	
Resting Time	
Sets Goal	
Completed ?	

❹ THURSDAY

1 2 3 4 5

EXERCISE & LEVEL   ① ② ③ ④ ⑤

Exercise Time	
Resting Time	
Sets Goal	
Completed ?	

❺ FRIDAY

1 2 3 4 5

Move on to the next step if you have completed five ticks in a row. ✓

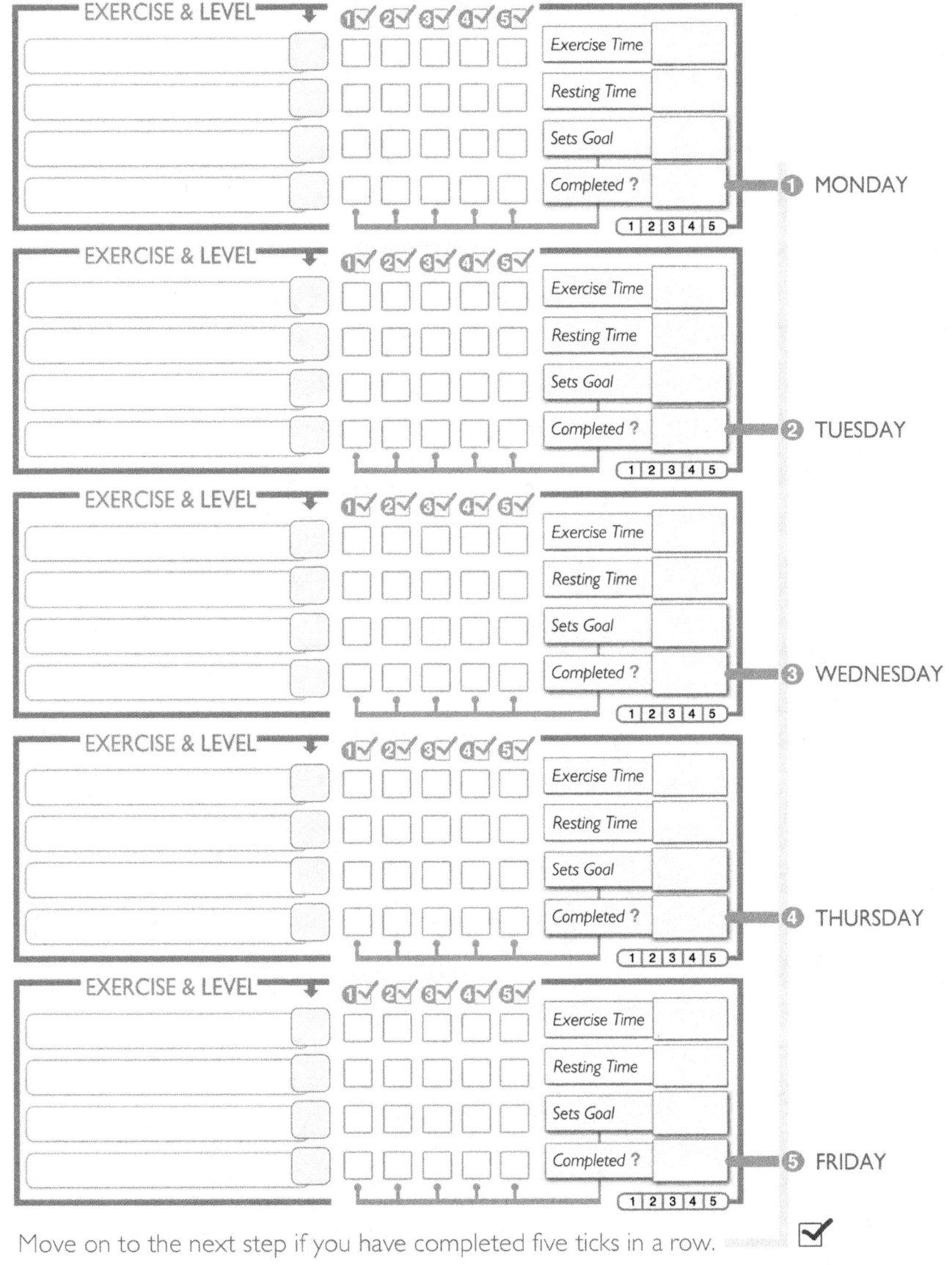

EXERCISE & LEVEL ① ✓ ② ✓ ③ ✓ ④ ✓ ⑤ ✓

Exercise Time
Resting Time
Sets Goal
Completed ?

❶ MONDAY

1 2 3 4 5

EXERCISE & LEVEL ① ✓ ② ✓ ③ ✓ ④ ✓ ⑤ ✓

Exercise Time
Resting Time
Sets Goal
Completed ?

❷ TUESDAY

1 2 3 4 5

EXERCISE & LEVEL ① ✓ ② ✓ ③ ✓ ④ ✓ ⑤ ✓

Exercise Time
Resting Time
Sets Goal
Completed ?

❸ WEDNESDAY

1 2 3 4 5

EXERCISE & LEVEL ① ✓ ② ✓ ③ ✓ ④ ✓ ⑤ ✓

Exercise Time
Resting Time
Sets Goal
Completed ?

❹ THURSDAY

1 2 3 4 5

EXERCISE & LEVEL ① ✓ ② ✓ ③ ✓ ④ ✓ ⑤ ✓

Exercise Time
Resting Time
Sets Goal
Completed ?

❺ FRIDAY

1 2 3 4 5

Move on to the next step if you have completed five ticks in a row. ☑

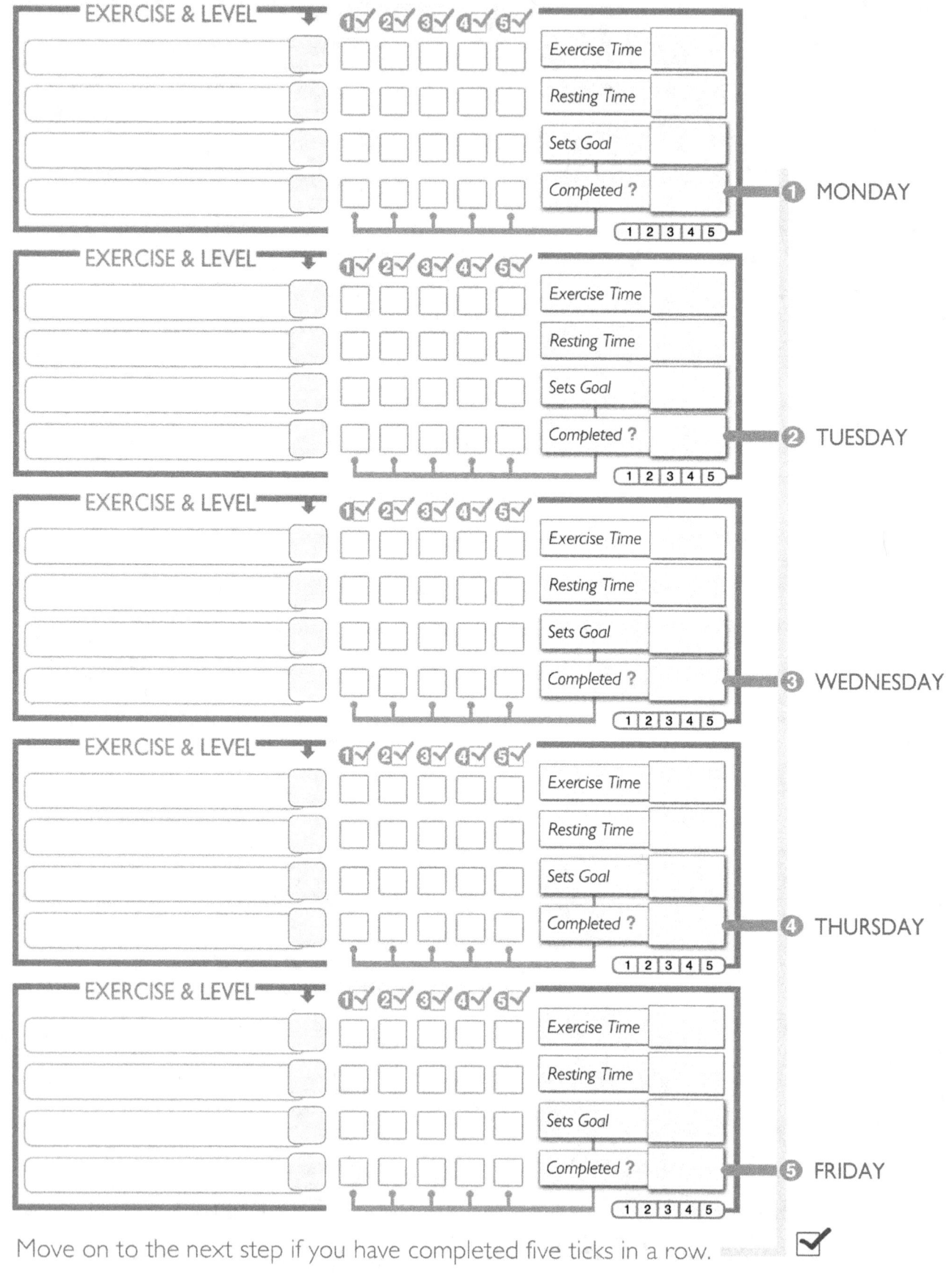

EXERCISE & LEVEL — 1 ✓ 2 ✓ 3 ✓ 4 ✓ 5 ✓

Exercise Time
Resting Time
Sets Goal
Completed ?
1 2 3 4 5

1 MONDAY

EXERCISE & LEVEL — 1 ✓ 2 ✓ 3 ✓ 4 ✓ 5 ✓

Exercise Time
Resting Time
Sets Goal
Completed ?
1 2 3 4 5

2 TUESDAY

EXERCISE & LEVEL — 1 ✓ 2 ✓ 3 ✓ 4 ✓ 5 ✓

Exercise Time
Resting Time
Sets Goal
Completed ?
1 2 3 4 5

3 WEDNESDAY

EXERCISE & LEVEL — 1 ✓ 2 ✓ 3 ✓ 4 ✓ 5 ✓

Exercise Time
Resting Time
Sets Goal
Completed ?
1 2 3 4 5

4 THURSDAY

EXERCISE & LEVEL — 1 ✓ 2 ✓ 3 ✓ 4 ✓ 5 ✓

Exercise Time
Resting Time
Sets Goal
Completed ?
1 2 3 4 5

5 FRIDAY

Move on to the next step if you have completed five ticks in a row. ✓

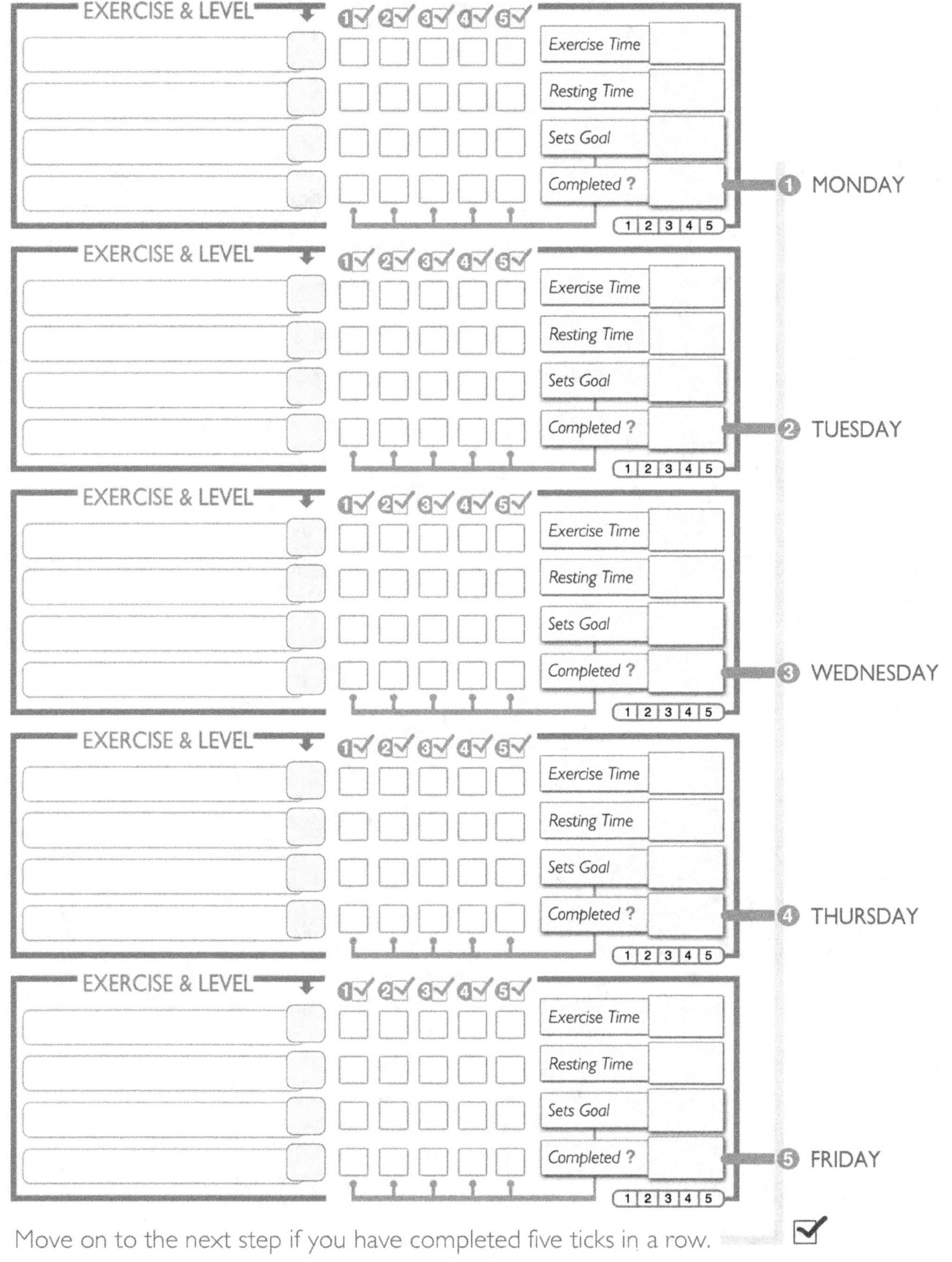

EXERCISE & LEVEL

① ② ③ ④ ⑤

Exercise Time

Resting Time

Sets Goal

Completed ?

1 2 3 4 5

1 MONDAY

EXERCISE & LEVEL

① ② ③ ④ ⑤

Exercise Time

Resting Time

Sets Goal

Completed ?

1 2 3 4 5

2 TUESDAY

EXERCISE & LEVEL

① ② ③ ④ ⑤

Exercise Time

Resting Time

Sets Goal

Completed ?

1 2 3 4 5

3 WEDNESDAY

EXERCISE & LEVEL

① ② ③ ④ ⑤

Exercise Time

Resting Time

Sets Goal

Completed ?

1 2 3 4 5

4 THURSDAY

EXERCISE & LEVEL

① ② ③ ④ ⑤

Exercise Time

Resting Time

Sets Goal

Completed ?

1 2 3 4 5

5 FRIDAY

Move on to the next step if you have completed five ticks in a row. ✓

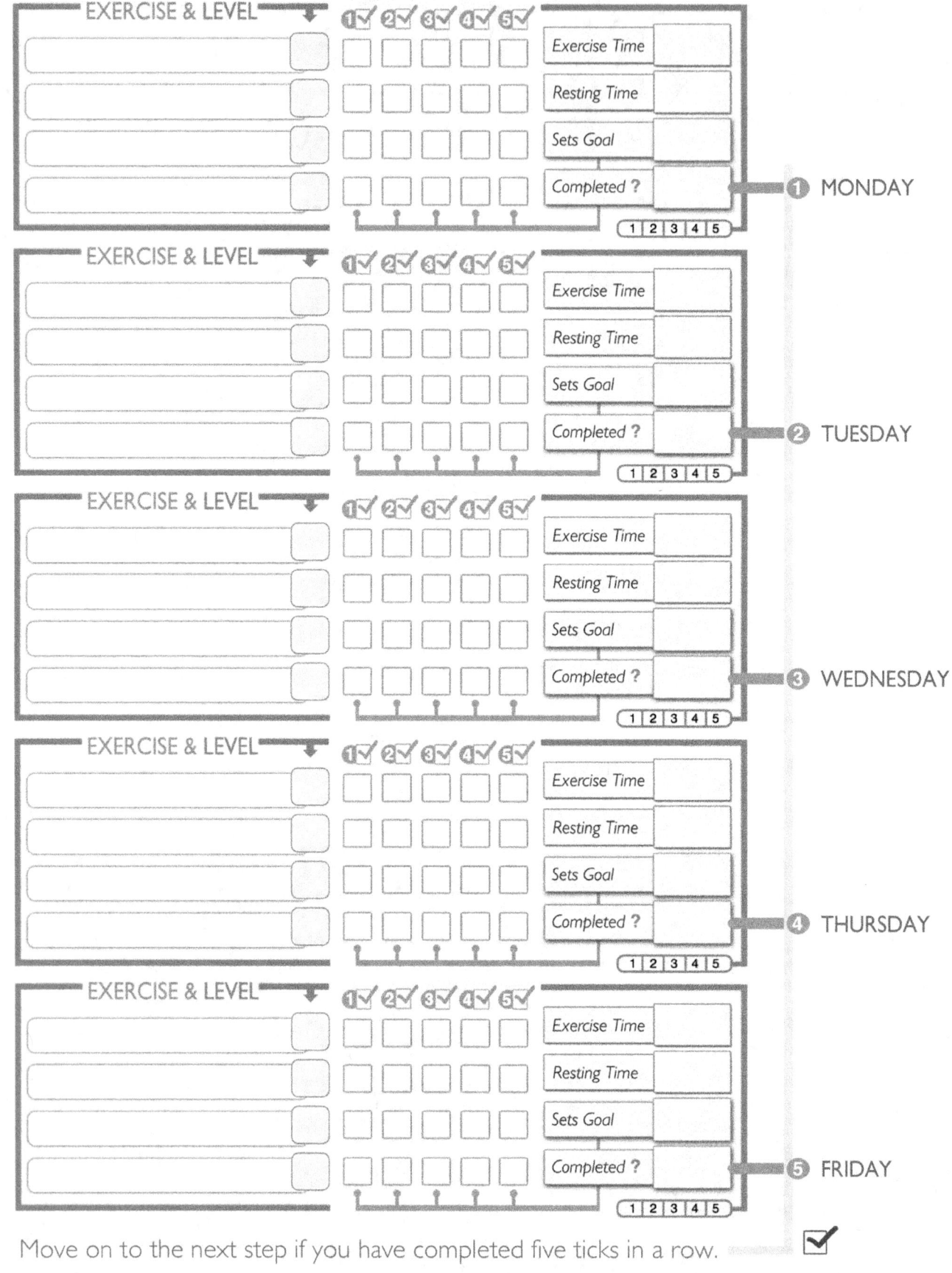

EXERCISE & LEVEL — 1✓ 2✓ 3✓ 4✓ 5✓

Exercise Time
Resting Time
Sets Goal
Completed ?
1 2 3 4 5

❶ MONDAY

EXERCISE & LEVEL — 1✓ 2✓ 3✓ 4✓ 5✓

Exercise Time
Resting Time
Sets Goal
Completed ?
1 2 3 4 5

❷ TUESDAY

EXERCISE & LEVEL — 1✓ 2✓ 3✓ 4✓ 5✓

Exercise Time
Resting Time
Sets Goal
Completed ?
1 2 3 4 5

❸ WEDNESDAY

EXERCISE & LEVEL — 1✓ 2✓ 3✓ 4✓ 5✓

Exercise Time
Resting Time
Sets Goal
Completed ?
1 2 3 4 5

❹ THURSDAY

EXERCISE & LEVEL — 1✓ 2✓ 3✓ 4✓ 5✓

Exercise Time
Resting Time
Sets Goal
Completed ?
1 2 3 4 5

❺ FRIDAY

Move on to the next step if you have completed five ticks in a row. ☑

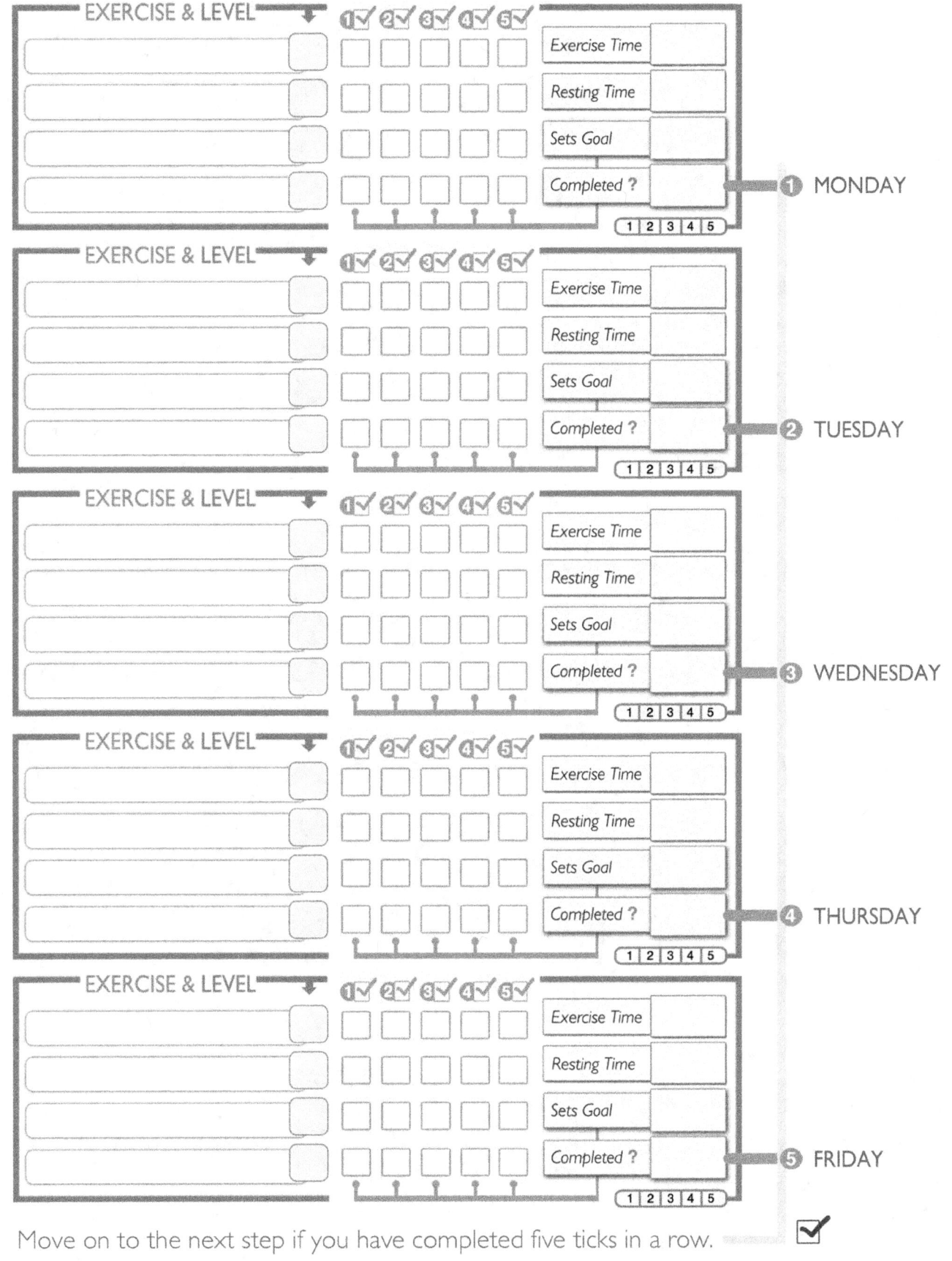

EXERCISE & LEVEL ☑1 ☑2 ☑3 ☑4 ☑5

Exercise Time
Resting Time
Sets Goal
Completed ?

❶ MONDAY

1 2 3 4 5

EXERCISE & LEVEL ☑1 ☑2 ☑3 ☑4 ☑5

Exercise Time
Resting Time
Sets Goal
Completed ?

❷ TUESDAY

1 2 3 4 5

EXERCISE & LEVEL ☑1 ☑2 ☑3 ☑4 ☑5

Exercise Time
Resting Time
Sets Goal
Completed ?

❸ WEDNESDAY

1 2 3 4 5

EXERCISE & LEVEL ☑1 ☑2 ☑3 ☑4 ☑5

Exercise Time
Resting Time
Sets Goal
Completed ?

❹ THURSDAY

1 2 3 4 5

EXERCISE & LEVEL ☑1 ☑2 ☑3 ☑4 ☑5

Exercise Time
Resting Time
Sets Goal
Completed ?

❺ FRIDAY

1 2 3 4 5

Move on to the next step if you have completed five ticks in a row. ☑

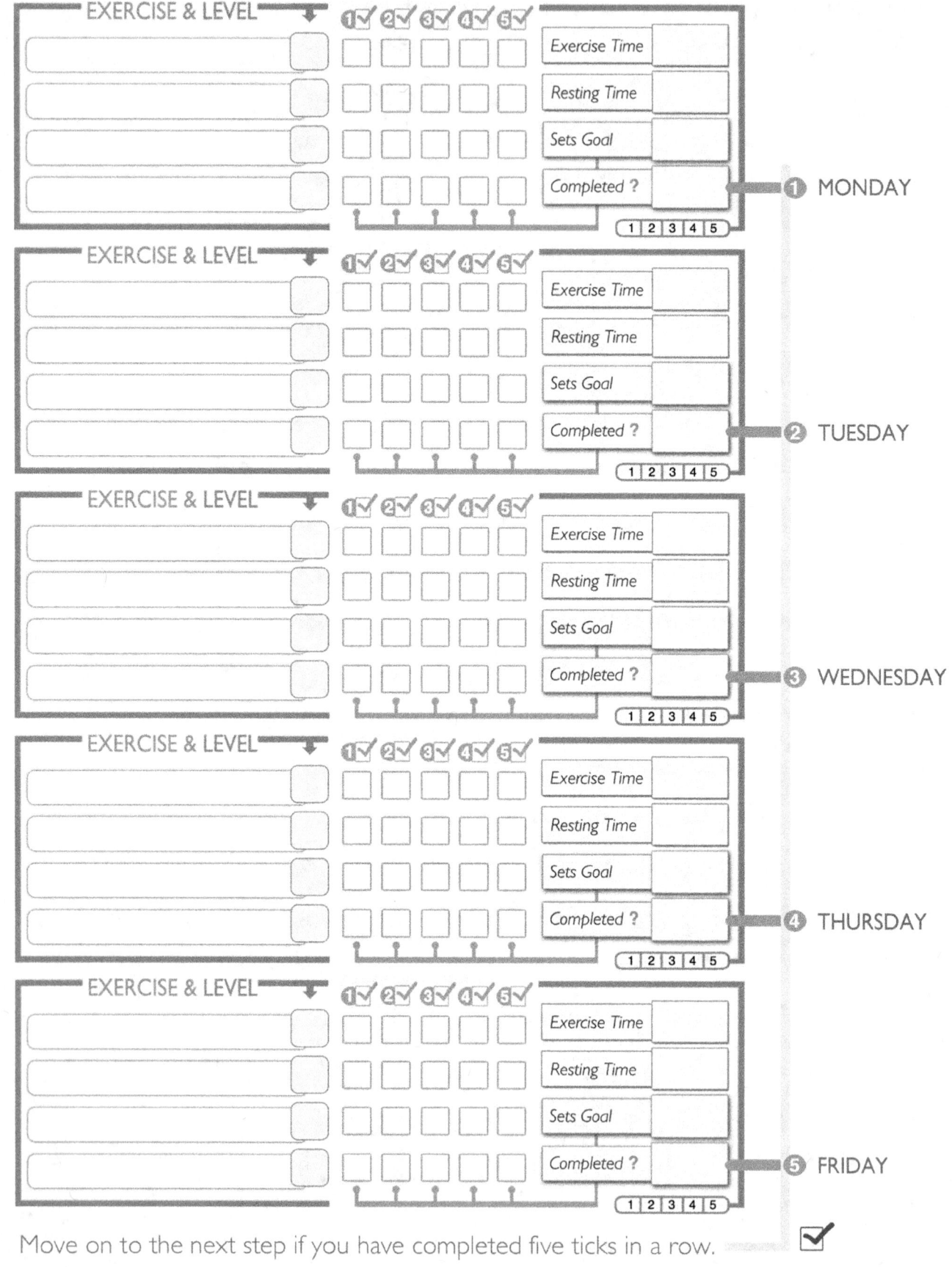

EXERCISE & LEVEL ① ② ③ ④ ⑤

① MONDAY

Exercise Time
Resting Time
Sets Goal
Completed ?

1 2 3 4 5

EXERCISE & LEVEL ① ② ③ ④ ⑤

② TUESDAY

Exercise Time
Resting Time
Sets Goal
Completed ?

1 2 3 4 5

EXERCISE & LEVEL ① ② ③ ④ ⑤

③ WEDNESDAY

Exercise Time
Resting Time
Sets Goal
Completed ?

1 2 3 4 5

EXERCISE & LEVEL ① ② ③ ④ ⑤

④ THURSDAY

Exercise Time
Resting Time
Sets Goal
Completed ?

1 2 3 4 5

EXERCISE & LEVEL ① ② ③ ④ ⑤

⑤ FRIDAY

Exercise Time
Resting Time
Sets Goal
Completed ?

1 2 3 4 5

Move on to the next step if you have completed five ticks in a row. ☑

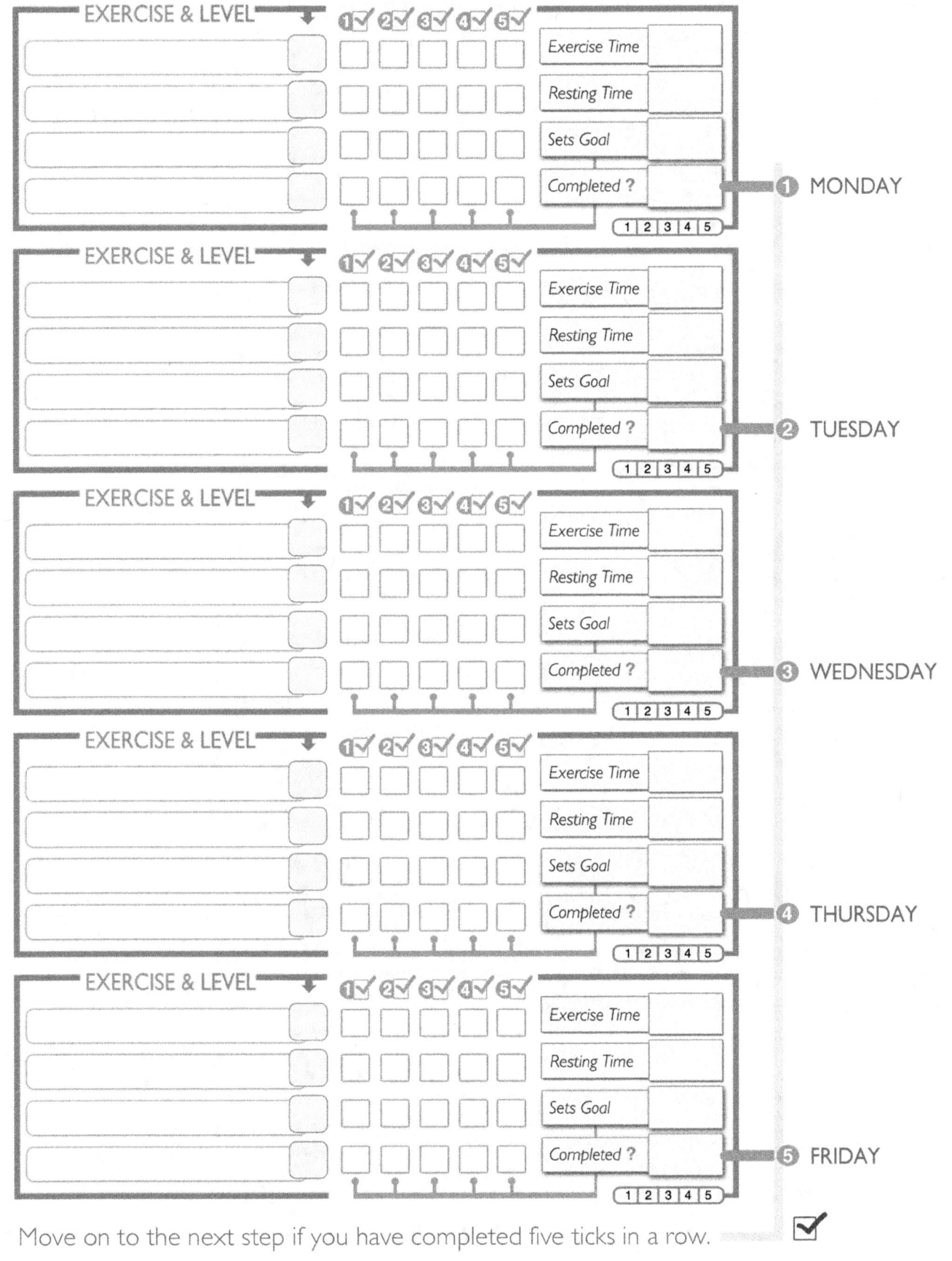

EXERCISE & LEVEL

1☑ 2☑ 3☑ 4☑ 5☑

Exercise Time
Resting Time
Sets Goal
Completed ?

① MONDAY

1 2 3 4 5

EXERCISE & LEVEL

1☑ 2☑ 3☑ 4☑ 5☑

Exercise Time
Resting Time
Sets Goal
Completed ?

② TUESDAY

1 2 3 4 5

EXERCISE & LEVEL

1☑ 2☑ 3☑ 4☑ 5☑

Exercise Time
Resting Time
Sets Goal
Completed ?

③ WEDNESDAY

1 2 3 4 5

EXERCISE & LEVEL

1☑ 2☑ 3☑ 4☑ 5☑

Exercise Time
Resting Time
Sets Goal
Completed ?

④ THURSDAY

1 2 3 4 5

EXERCISE & LEVEL

1☑ 2☑ 3☑ 4☑ 5☑

Exercise Time
Resting Time
Sets Goal
Completed ?

⑤ FRIDAY

1 2 3 4 5

Move on to the next step if you have completed five ticks in a row. ☑

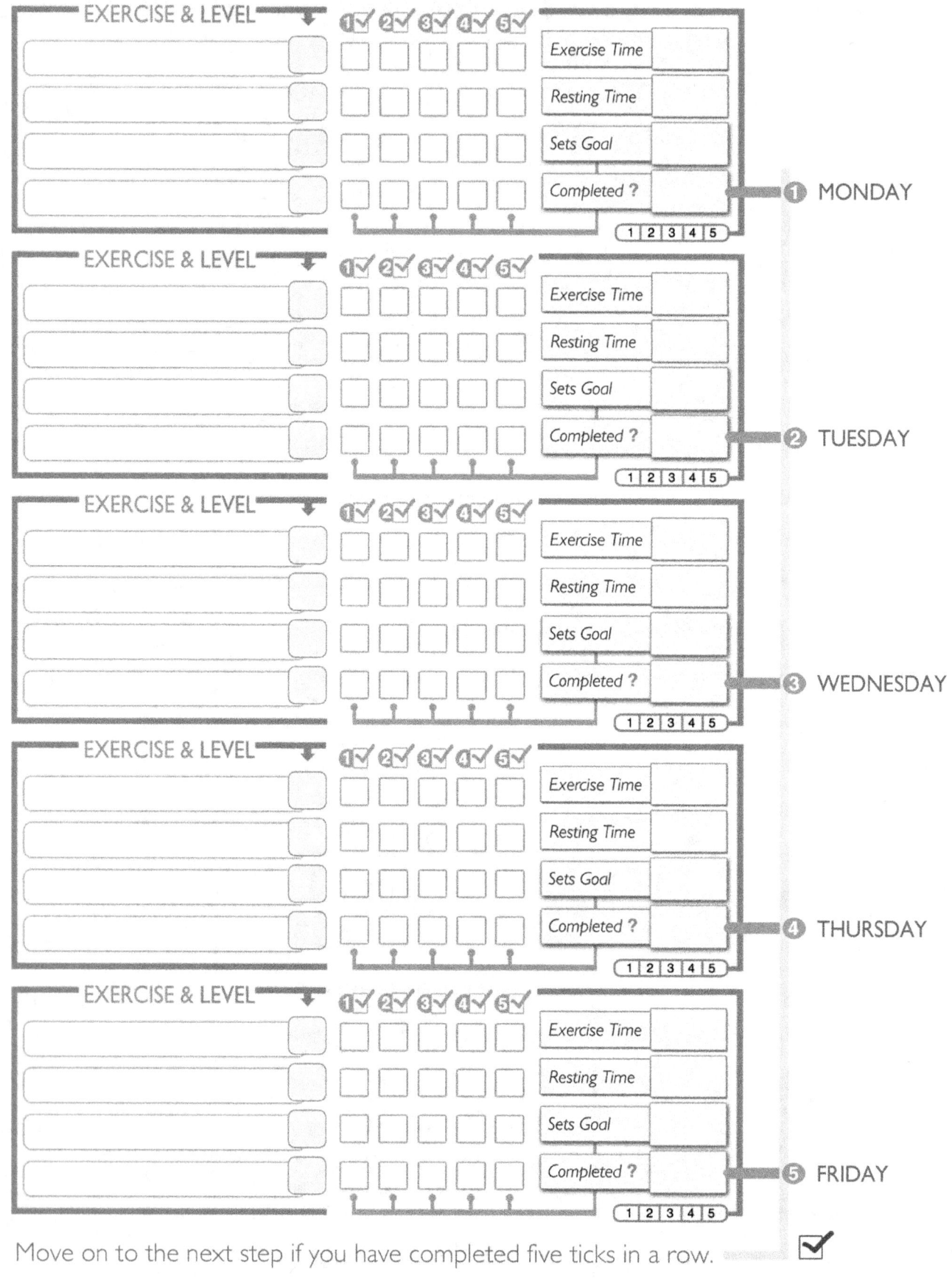

EXERCISE & LEVEL 1 2 3 4 5

Exercise Time

Resting Time

Sets Goal

Completed ? 1 2 3 4 5

① MONDAY

EXERCISE & LEVEL 1 2 3 4 5

Exercise Time

Resting Time

Sets Goal

Completed ? 1 2 3 4 5

② TUESDAY

EXERCISE & LEVEL 1 2 3 4 5

Exercise Time

Resting Time

Sets Goal

Completed ? 1 2 3 4 5

③ WEDNESDAY

EXERCISE & LEVEL 1 2 3 4 5

Exercise Time

Resting Time

Sets Goal

Completed ? 1 2 3 4 5

④ THURSDAY

EXERCISE & LEVEL 1 2 3 4 5

Exercise Time

Resting Time

Sets Goal

Completed ? 1 2 3 4 5

⑤ FRIDAY

Move on to the next step if you have completed five ticks in a row.

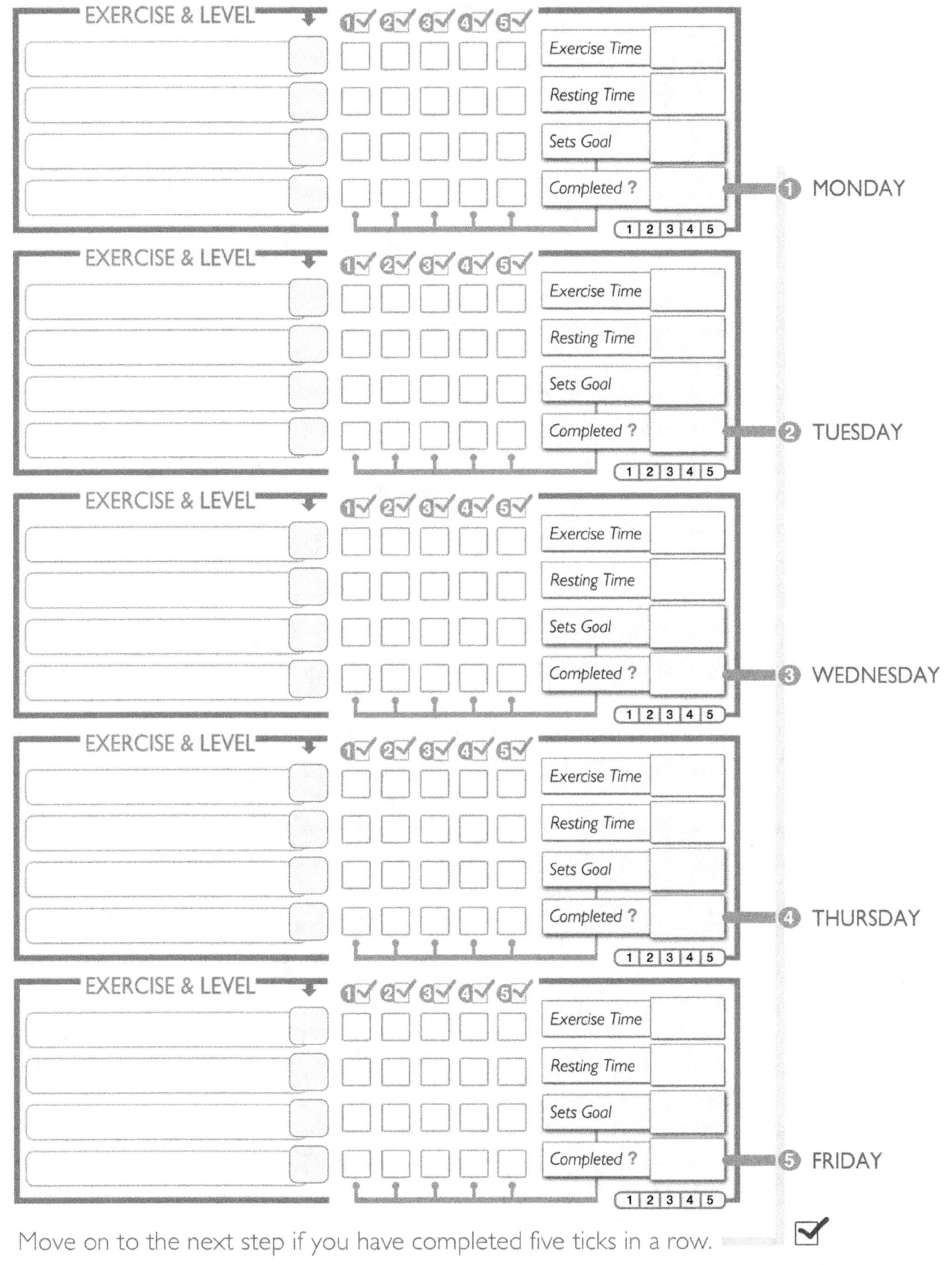

EXERCISE & LEVEL ▼　1✓ 2✓ 3✓ 4✓ 5✓

Exercise Time

Resting Time

Sets Goal

Completed ? ━━● ① MONDAY

`1 2 3 4 5`

EXERCISE & LEVEL ▼　1✓ 2✓ 3✓ 4✓ 5✓

Exercise Time

Resting Time

Sets Goal

Completed ? ━━● ② TUESDAY

`1 2 3 4 5`

EXERCISE & LEVEL ▼　1✓ 2✓ 3✓ 4✓ 5✓

Exercise Time

Resting Time

Sets Goal

Completed ? ━━● ③ WEDNESDAY

`1 2 3 4 5`

EXERCISE & LEVEL ▼　1✓ 2✓ 3✓ 4✓ 5✓

Exercise Time

Resting Time

Sets Goal

Completed ? ━━● ④ THURSDAY

`1 2 3 4 5`

EXERCISE & LEVEL ▼　1✓ 2✓ 3✓ 4✓ 5✓

Exercise Time

Resting Time

Sets Goal

Completed ? ━━● ⑤ FRIDAY

`1 2 3 4 5`

Move on to the next step if you have completed five ticks in a row. ☑

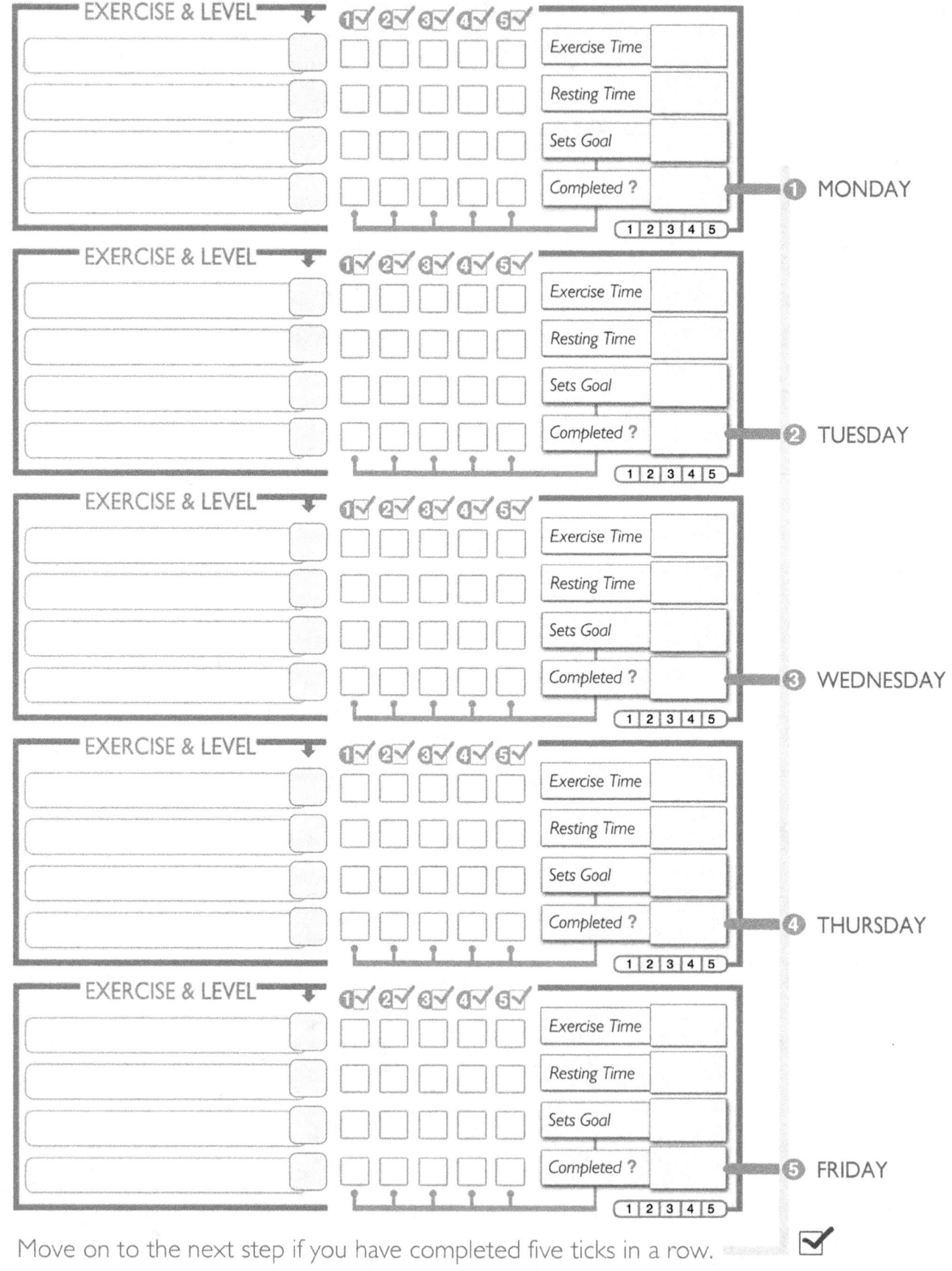

EXERCISE & LEVEL

1☑ 2☑ 3☑ 4☑ 5☑

Exercise Time

Resting Time

Sets Goal

Completed ?

1 2 3 4 5

1 MONDAY

EXERCISE & LEVEL

1☑ 2☑ 3☑ 4☑ 5☑

Exercise Time

Resting Time

Sets Goal

Completed ?

1 2 3 4 5

2 TUESDAY

EXERCISE & LEVEL

1☑ 2☑ 3☑ 4☑ 5☑

Exercise Time

Resting Time

Sets Goal

Completed ?

1 2 3 4 5

3 WEDNESDAY

EXERCISE & LEVEL

1☑ 2☑ 3☑ 4☑ 5☑

Exercise Time

Resting Time

Sets Goal

Completed ?

1 2 3 4 5

4 THURSDAY

EXERCISE & LEVEL

1☑ 2☑ 3☑ 4☑ 5☑

Exercise Time

Resting Time

Sets Goal

Completed ?

1 2 3 4 5

5 FRIDAY

Move on to the next step if you have completed five ticks in a row. ☑

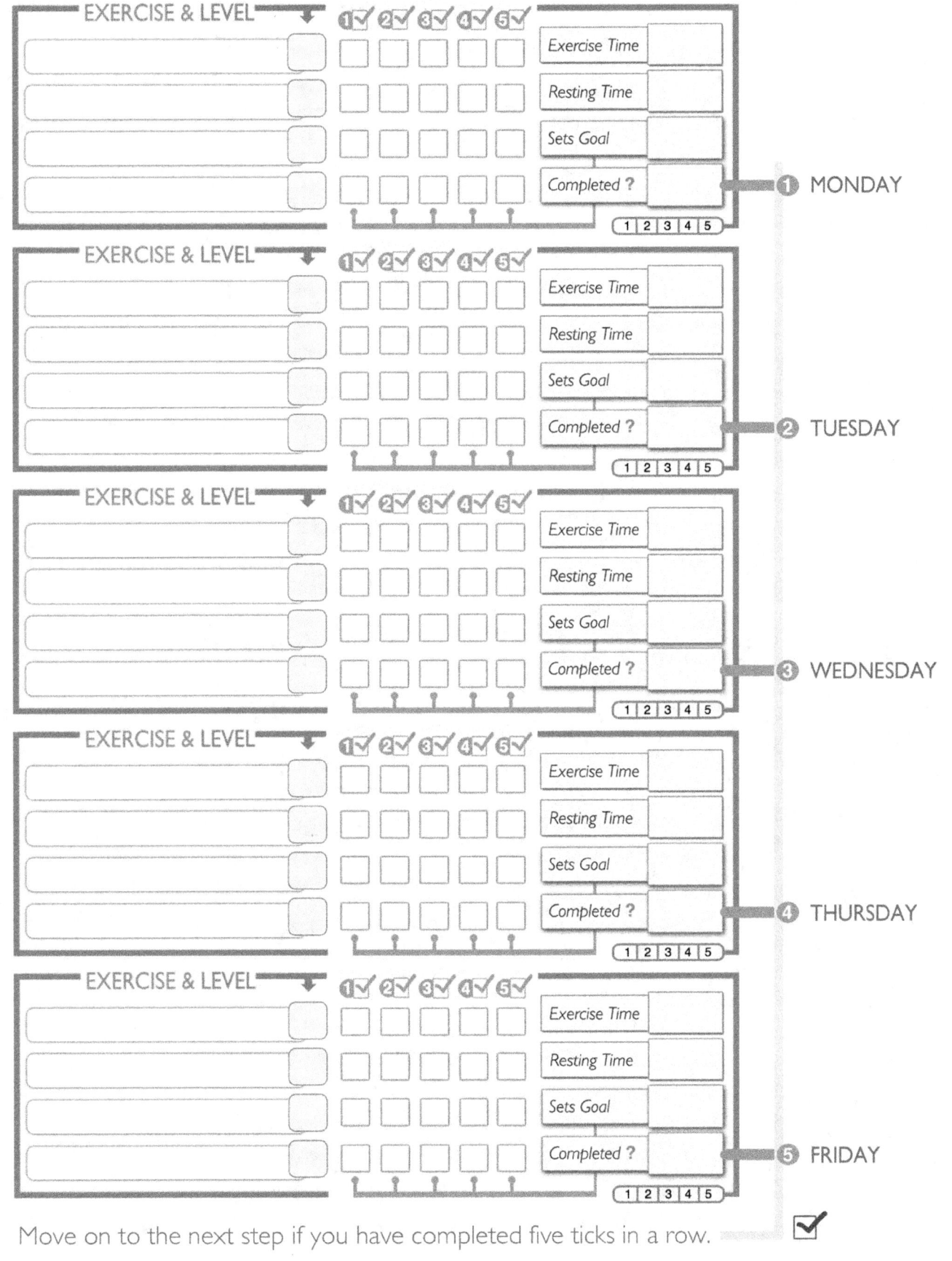

EXERCISE & LEVEL	1 ✓ 2 ✓ 3 ✓ 4 ✓ 5 ✓				

Exercise Time
Resting Time
Sets Goal
Completed ?
1 2 3 4 5

① MONDAY

Exercise Time
Resting Time
Sets Goal
Completed ?
1 2 3 4 5

② TUESDAY

Exercise Time
Resting Time
Sets Goal
Completed ?
1 2 3 4 5

③ WEDNESDAY

Exercise Time
Resting Time
Sets Goal
Completed ?
1 2 3 4 5

④ THURSDAY

Exercise Time
Resting Time
Sets Goal
Completed ?
1 2 3 4 5

⑤ FRIDAY

Move on to the next step if you have completed five ticks in a row.

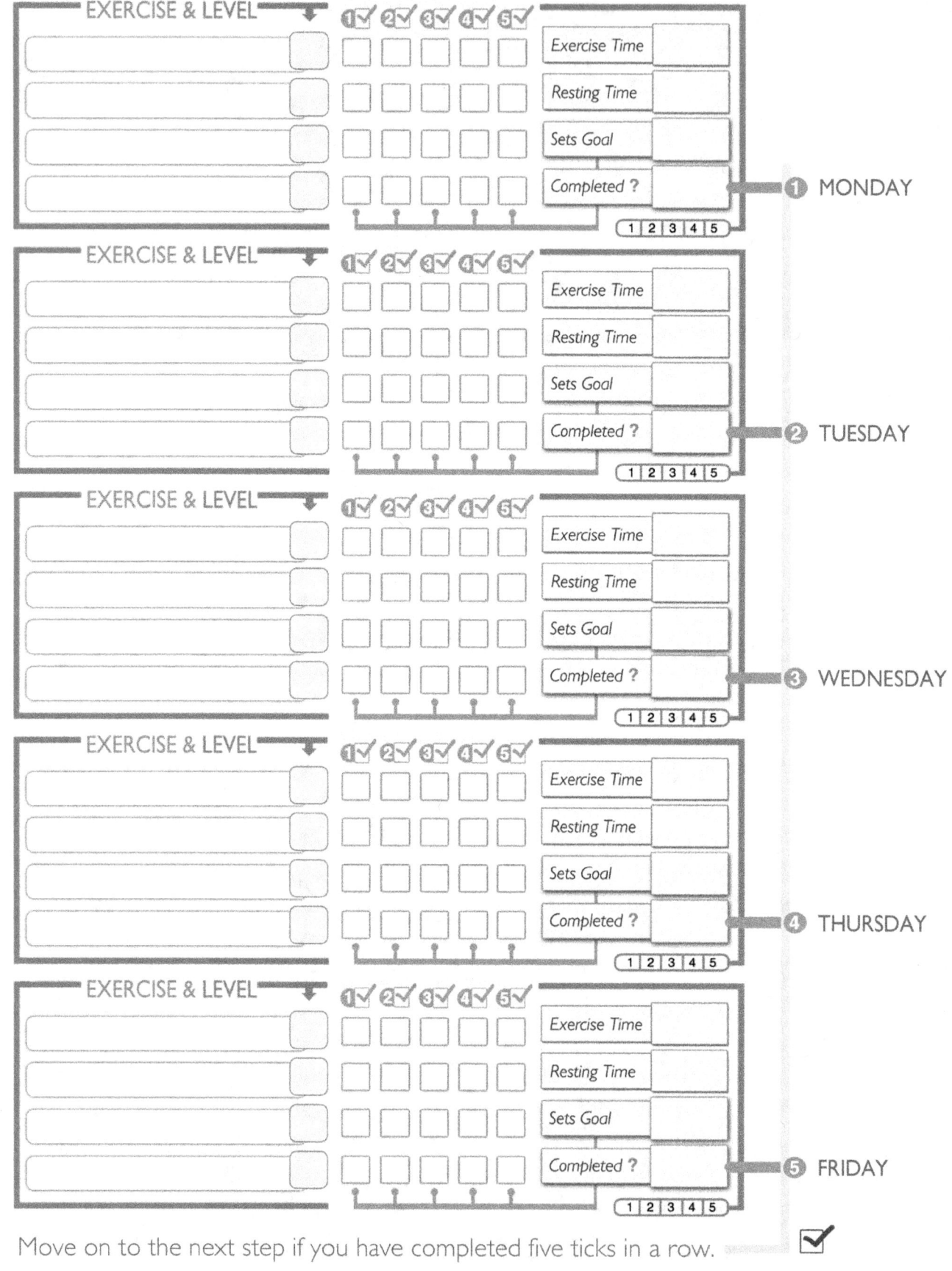

EXERCISE & LEVEL

1✓ 2✓ 3✓ 4✓ 5✓

Exercise Time
Resting Time
Sets Goal
Completed ?

1 2 3 4 5

❶ MONDAY

EXERCISE & LEVEL

1✓ 2✓ 3✓ 4✓ 5✓

Exercise Time
Resting Time
Sets Goal
Completed ?

1 2 3 4 5

❷ TUESDAY

EXERCISE & LEVEL

1✓ 2✓ 3✓ 4✓ 5✓

Exercise Time
Resting Time
Sets Goal
Completed ?

1 2 3 4 5

❸ WEDNESDAY

EXERCISE & LEVEL

1✓ 2✓ 3✓ 4✓ 5✓

Exercise Time
Resting Time
Sets Goal
Completed ?

1 2 3 4 5

❹ THURSDAY

EXERCISE & LEVEL

1✓ 2✓ 3✓ 4✓ 5✓

Exercise Time
Resting Time
Sets Goal
Completed ?

1 2 3 4 5

❺ FRIDAY

Move on to the next step if you have completed five ticks in a row. ☑

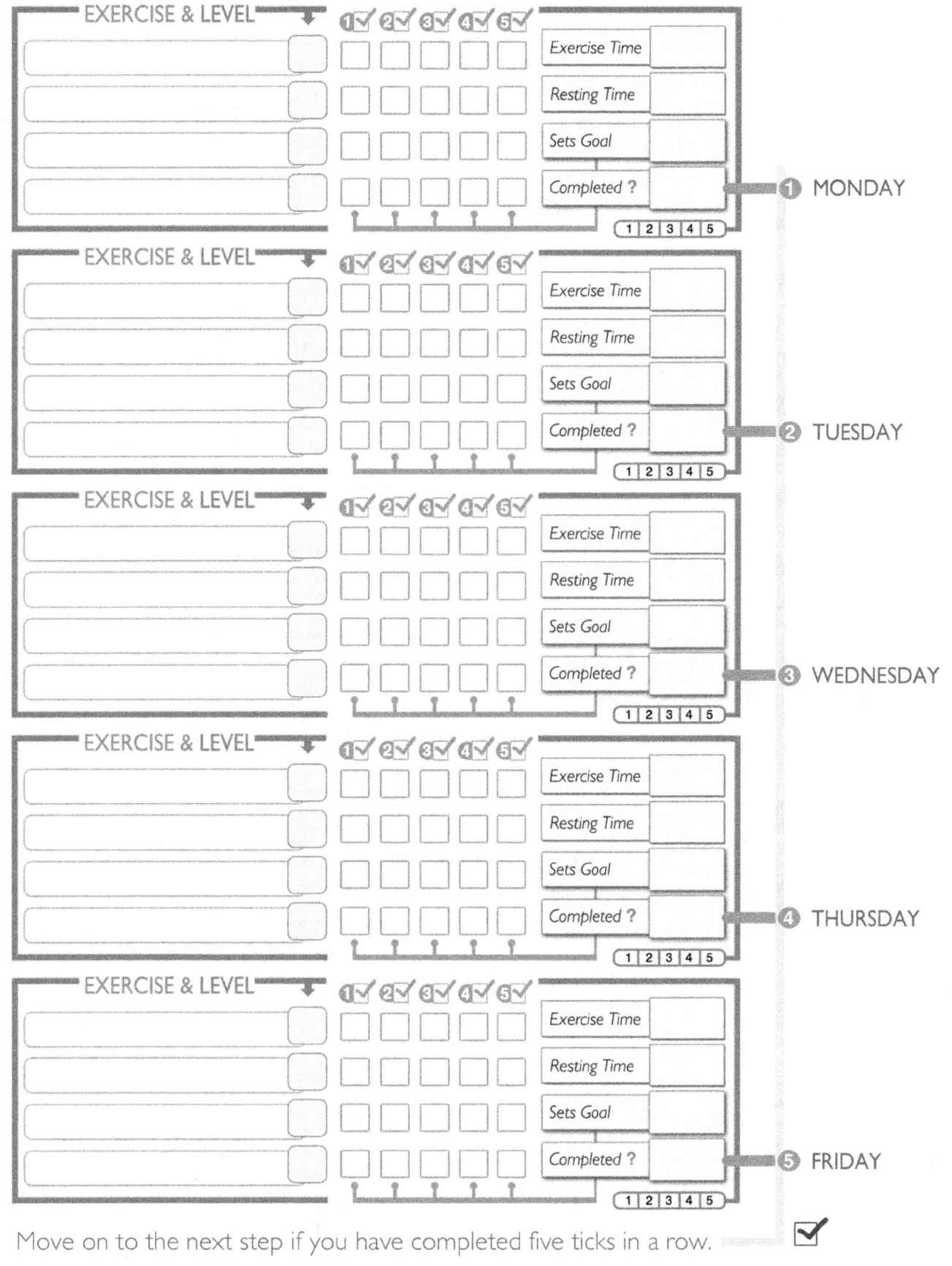

EXERCISE & LEVEL

① ② ③ ④ ⑤

Exercise Time
Resting Time
Sets Goal
Completed ?

1 2 3 4 5

① MONDAY

② TUESDAY

③ WEDNESDAY

④ THURSDAY

⑤ FRIDAY

Move on to the next step if you have completed five ticks in a row. ☑

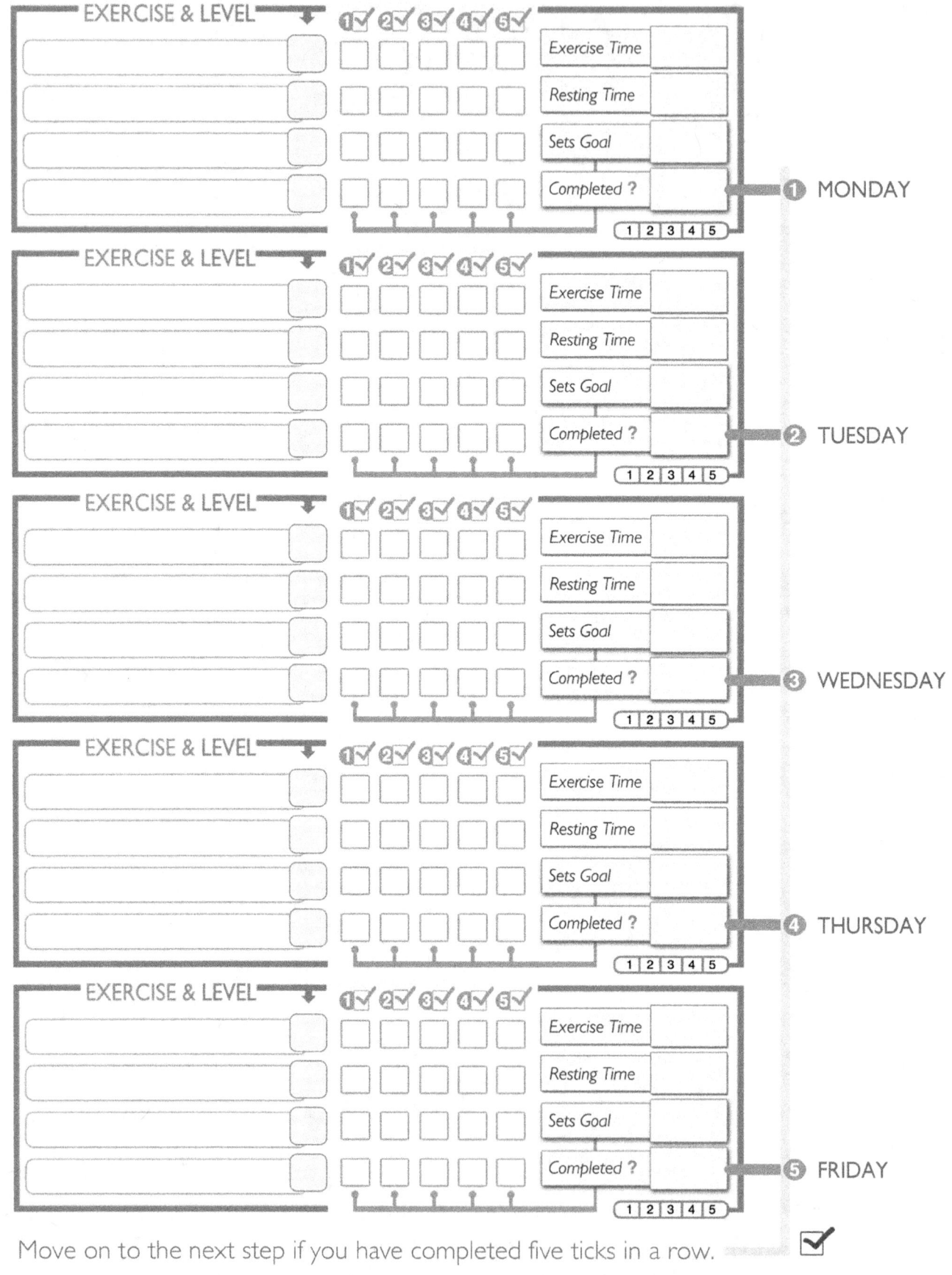

EXERCISE & LEVEL ▼ ①✓ ②✓ ③✓ ④✓ ⑤✓

Exercise Time

Resting Time

Sets Goal

Completed ?   1 2 3 4 5

❶ MONDAY

EXERCISE & LEVEL ▼ ①✓ ②✓ ③✓ ④✓ ⑤✓

Exercise Time

Resting Time

Sets Goal

Completed ?   1 2 3 4 5

❷ TUESDAY

EXERCISE & LEVEL ▼ ①✓ ②✓ ③✓ ④✓ ⑤✓

Exercise Time

Resting Time

Sets Goal

Completed ?   1 2 3 4 5

❸ WEDNESDAY

EXERCISE & LEVEL ▼ ①✓ ②✓ ③✓ ④✓ ⑤✓

Exercise Time

Resting Time

Sets Goal

Completed ?   1 2 3 4 5

❹ THURSDAY

EXERCISE & LEVEL ▼ ①✓ ②✓ ③✓ ④✓ ⑤✓

Exercise Time

Resting Time

Sets Goal

Completed ?   1 2 3 4 5

❺ FRIDAY

Move on to the next step if you have completed five ticks in a row. ✓

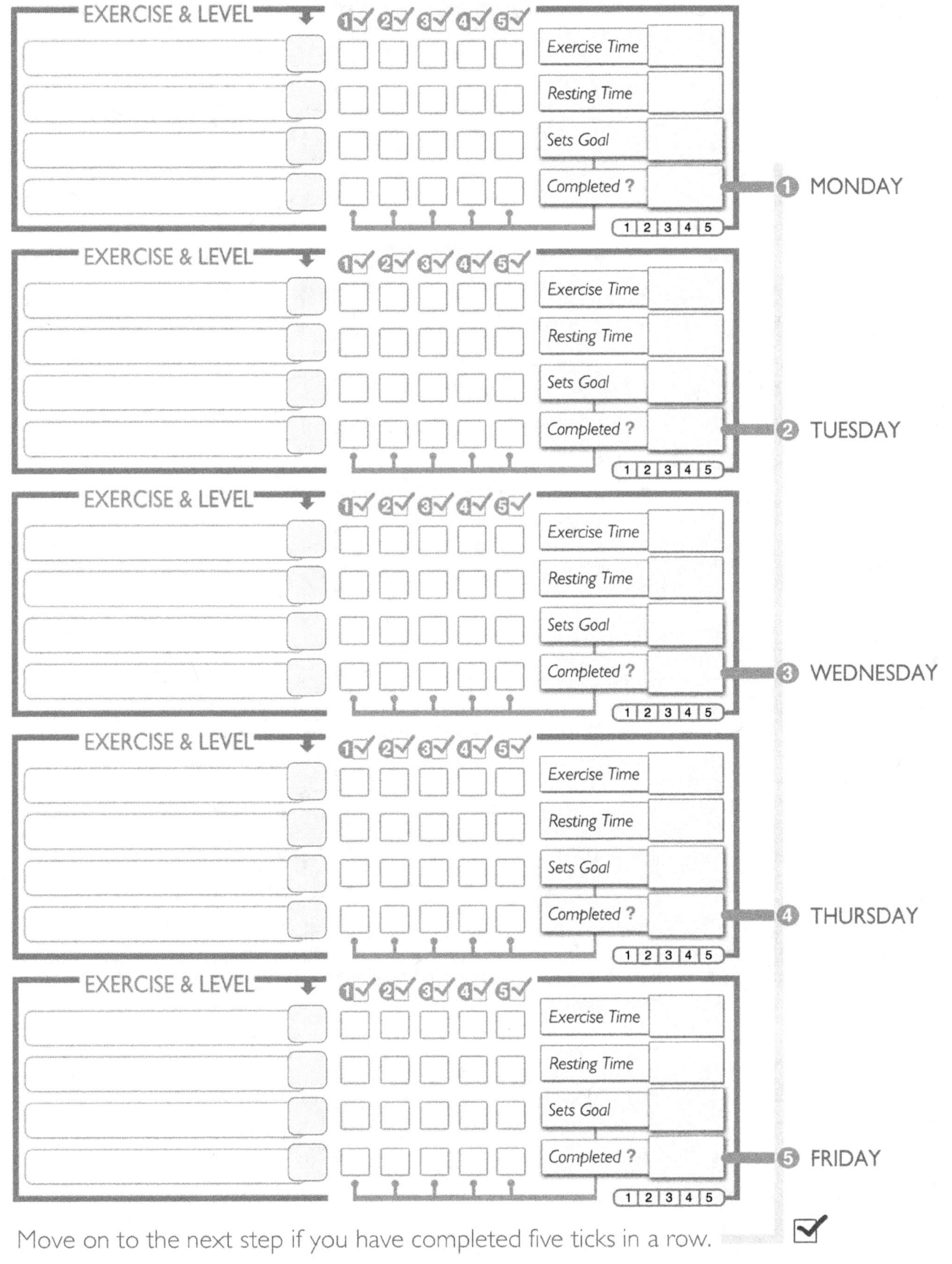

Move on to the next step if you have completed five ticks in a row.

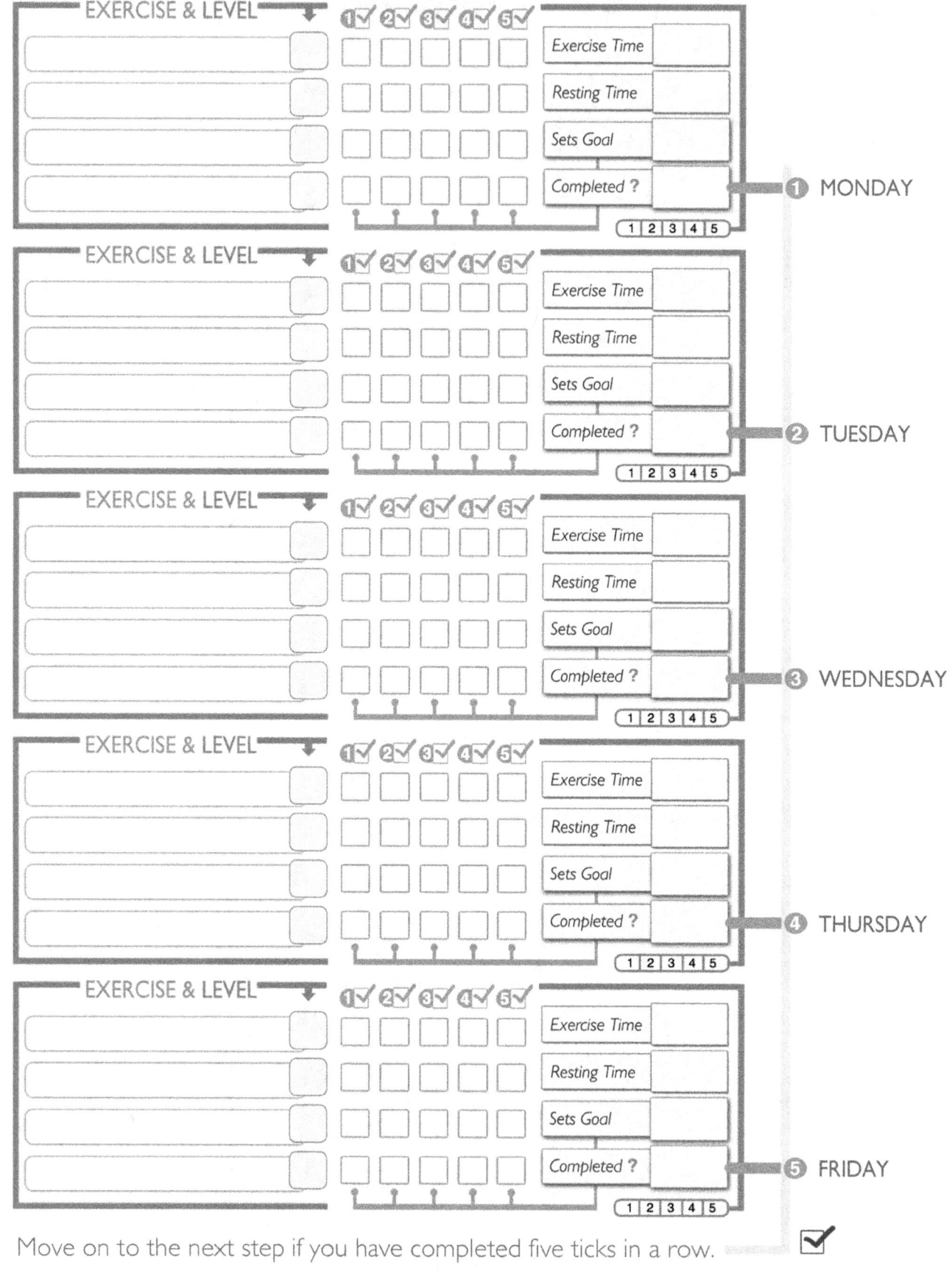

EXERCISE & LEVEL 1✓ 2✓ 3✓ 4✓ 5✓

Exercise Time

Resting Time

Sets Goal

Completed ?

① MONDAY

1 2 3 4 5

EXERCISE & LEVEL 1✓ 2✓ 3✓ 4✓ 5✓

Exercise Time

Resting Time

Sets Goal

Completed ?

② TUESDAY

1 2 3 4 5

EXERCISE & LEVEL 1✓ 2✓ 3✓ 4✓ 5✓

Exercise Time

Resting Time

Sets Goal

Completed ?

③ WEDNESDAY

1 2 3 4 5

EXERCISE & LEVEL 1✓ 2✓ 3✓ 4✓ 5✓

Exercise Time

Resting Time

Sets Goal

Completed ?

④ THURSDAY

1 2 3 4 5

EXERCISE & LEVEL 1✓ 2✓ 3✓ 4✓ 5✓

Exercise Time

Resting Time

Sets Goal

Completed ?

⑤ FRIDAY

1 2 3 4 5

Move on to the next step if you have completed five ticks in a row. ✓

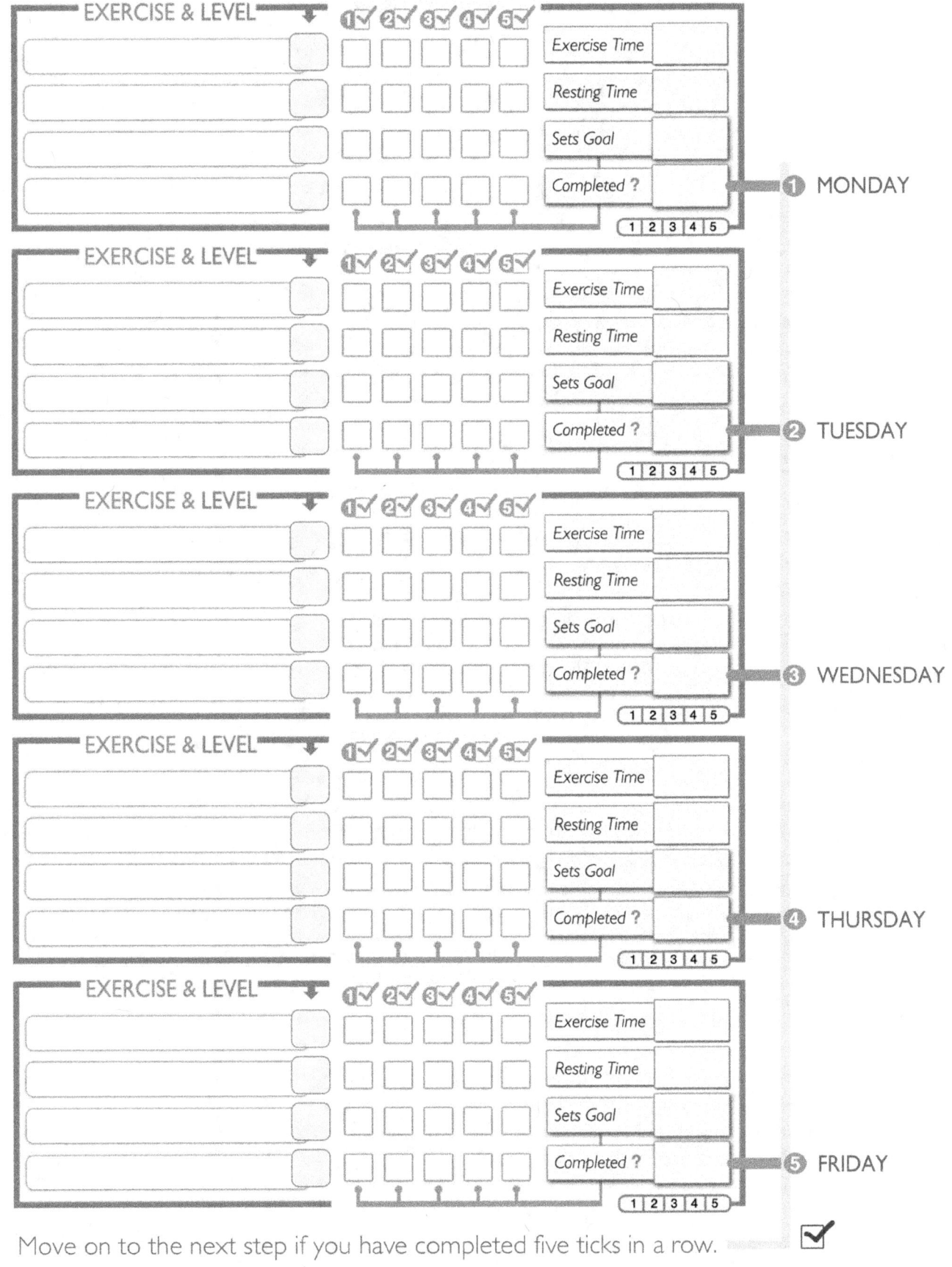

EXERCISE & LEVEL ① ② ③ ④ ⑤

Exercise Time

Resting Time

Sets Goal

Completed ?

❶ MONDAY

1 2 3 4 5

EXERCISE & LEVEL ① ② ③ ④ ⑤

Exercise Time

Resting Time

Sets Goal

Completed ?

❷ TUESDAY

1 2 3 4 5

EXERCISE & LEVEL ① ② ③ ④ ⑤

Exercise Time

Resting Time

Sets Goal

Completed ?

❸ WEDNESDAY

1 2 3 4 5

EXERCISE & LEVEL ① ② ③ ④ ⑤

Exercise Time

Resting Time

Sets Goal

Completed ?

❹ THURSDAY

1 2 3 4 5

EXERCISE & LEVEL ① ② ③ ④ ⑤

Exercise Time

Resting Time

Sets Goal

Completed ?

❺ FRIDAY

1 2 3 4 5

Move on to the next step if you have completed five ticks in a row. ☑

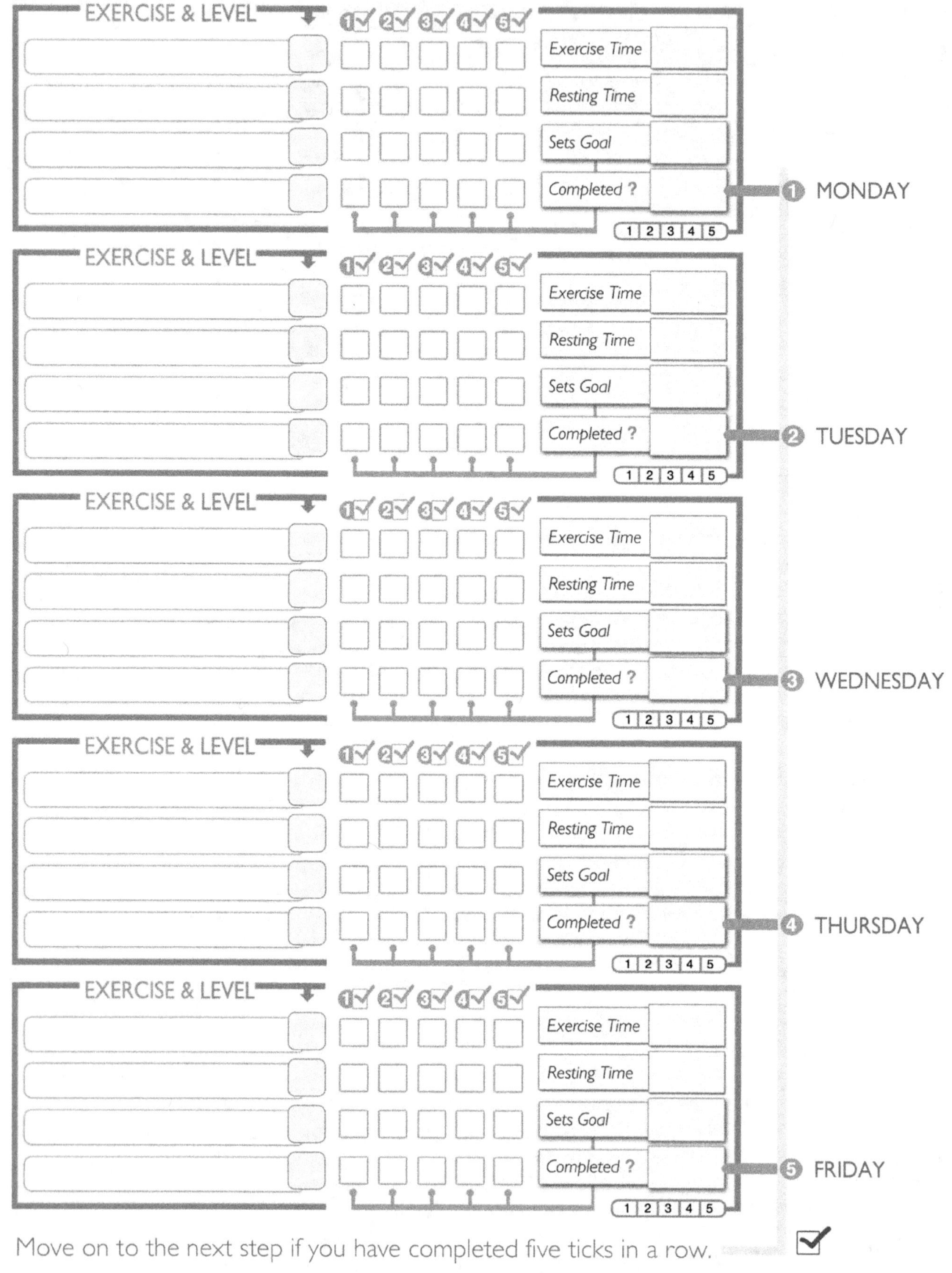

EXERCISE & LEVEL

1✓ 2✓ 3✓ 4✓ 5✓

Exercise Time

Resting Time

Sets Goal

Completed ?

1 MONDAY

1 2 3 4 5

EXERCISE & LEVEL

1✓ 2✓ 3✓ 4✓ 5✓

Exercise Time

Resting Time

Sets Goal

Completed ?

2 TUESDAY

1 2 3 4 5

EXERCISE & LEVEL

1✓ 2✓ 3✓ 4✓ 5✓

Exercise Time

Resting Time

Sets Goal

Completed ?

3 WEDNESDAY

1 2 3 4 5

EXERCISE & LEVEL

1✓ 2✓ 3✓ 4✓ 5✓

Exercise Time

Resting Time

Sets Goal

Completed ?

4 THURSDAY

1 2 3 4 5

EXERCISE & LEVEL

1✓ 2✓ 3✓ 4✓ 5✓

Exercise Time

Resting Time

Sets Goal

Completed ?

5 FRIDAY

1 2 3 4 5

Move on to the next step if you have completed five ticks in a row. ☑

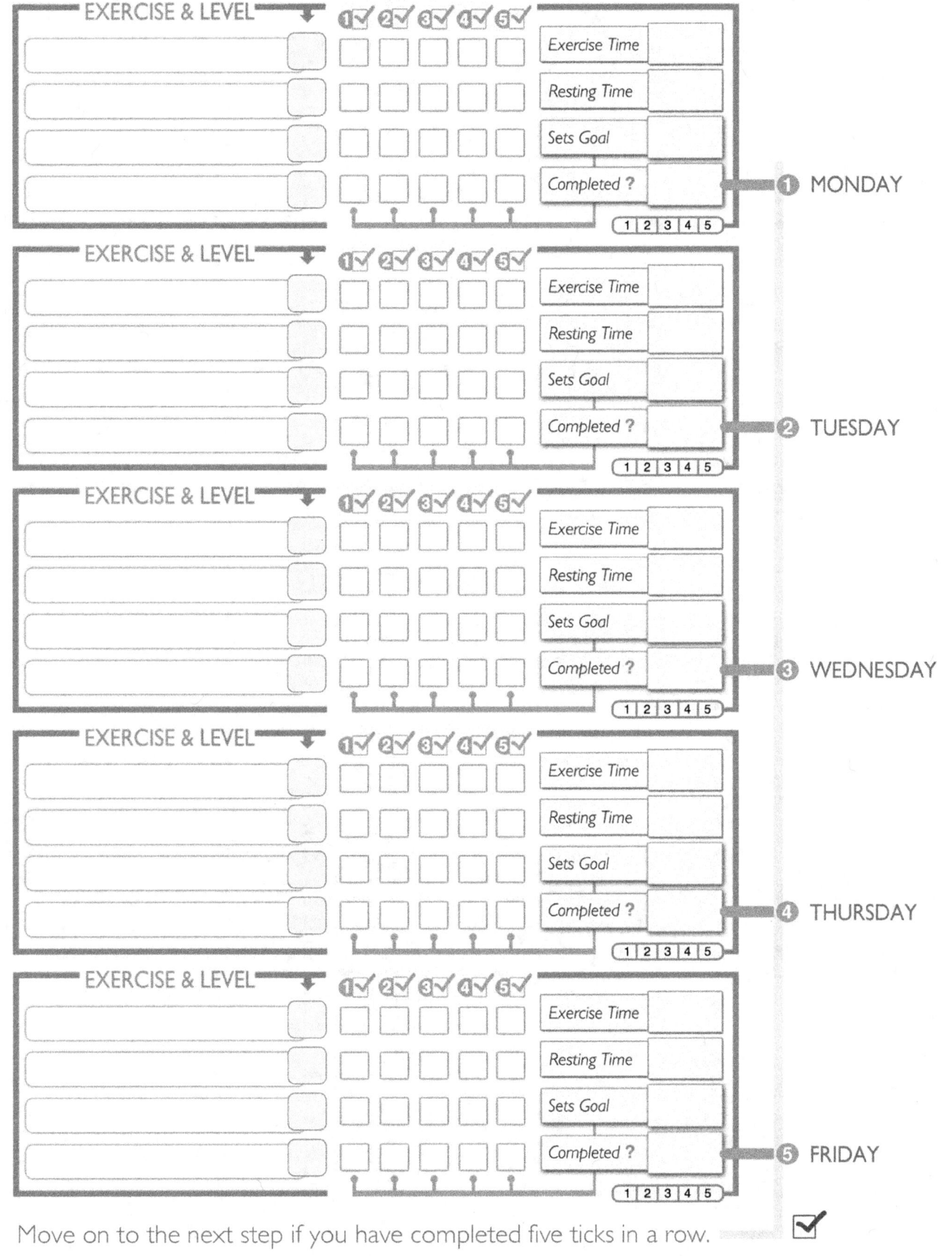

EXERCISE & LEVEL ❶✓ ❷✓ ❸✓ ❹✓ ❺✓

Exercise Time
Resting Time
Sets Goal
Completed ?

❶ MONDAY

1 2 3 4 5

EXERCISE & LEVEL ❶✓ ❷✓ ❸✓ ❹✓ ❺✓

Exercise Time
Resting Time
Sets Goal
Completed ?

❷ TUESDAY

1 2 3 4 5

EXERCISE & LEVEL ❶✓ ❷✓ ❸✓ ❹✓ ❺✓

Exercise Time
Resting Time
Sets Goal
Completed ?

❸ WEDNESDAY

1 2 3 4 5

EXERCISE & LEVEL ❶✓ ❷✓ ❸✓ ❹✓ ❺✓

Exercise Time
Resting Time
Sets Goal
Completed ?

❹ THURSDAY

1 2 3 4 5

EXERCISE & LEVEL ❶✓ ❷✓ ❸✓ ❹✓ ❺✓

Exercise Time
Resting Time
Sets Goal
Completed ?

❺ FRIDAY

1 2 3 4 5

Move on to the next step if you have completed five ticks in a row. ☑

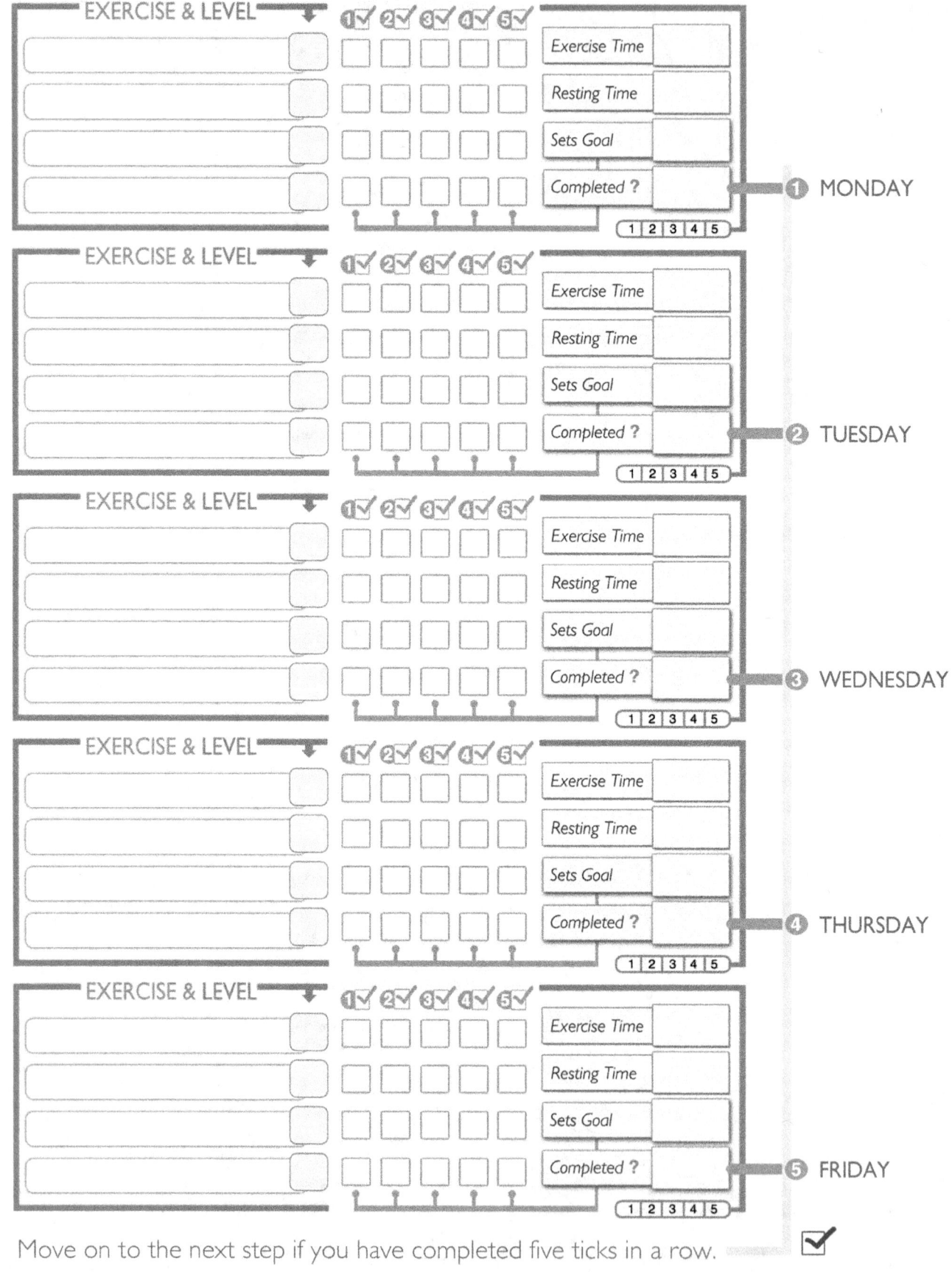

Move on to the next step if you have completed five ticks in a row. ☑

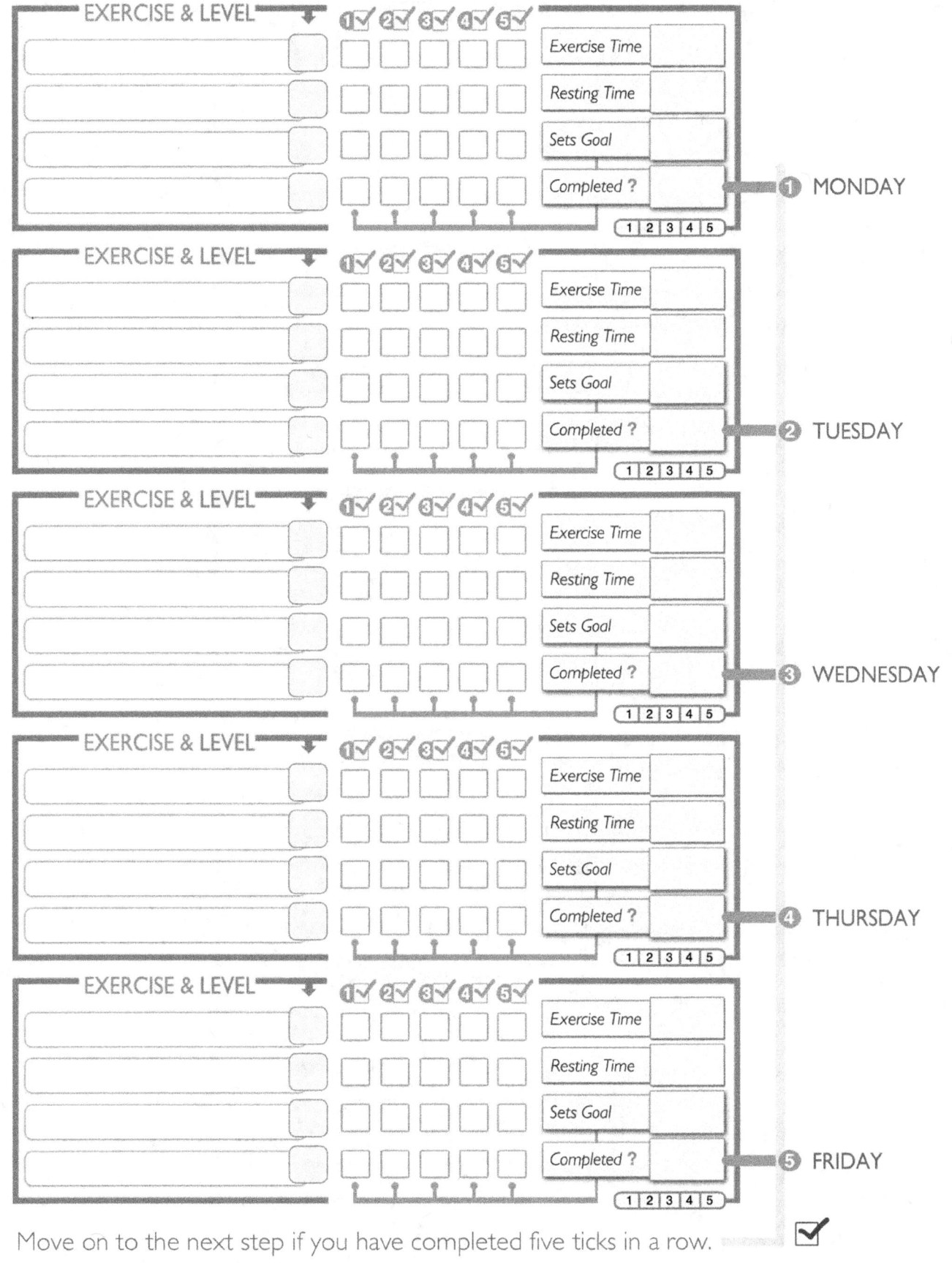

Move on to the next step if you have completed five ticks in a row.

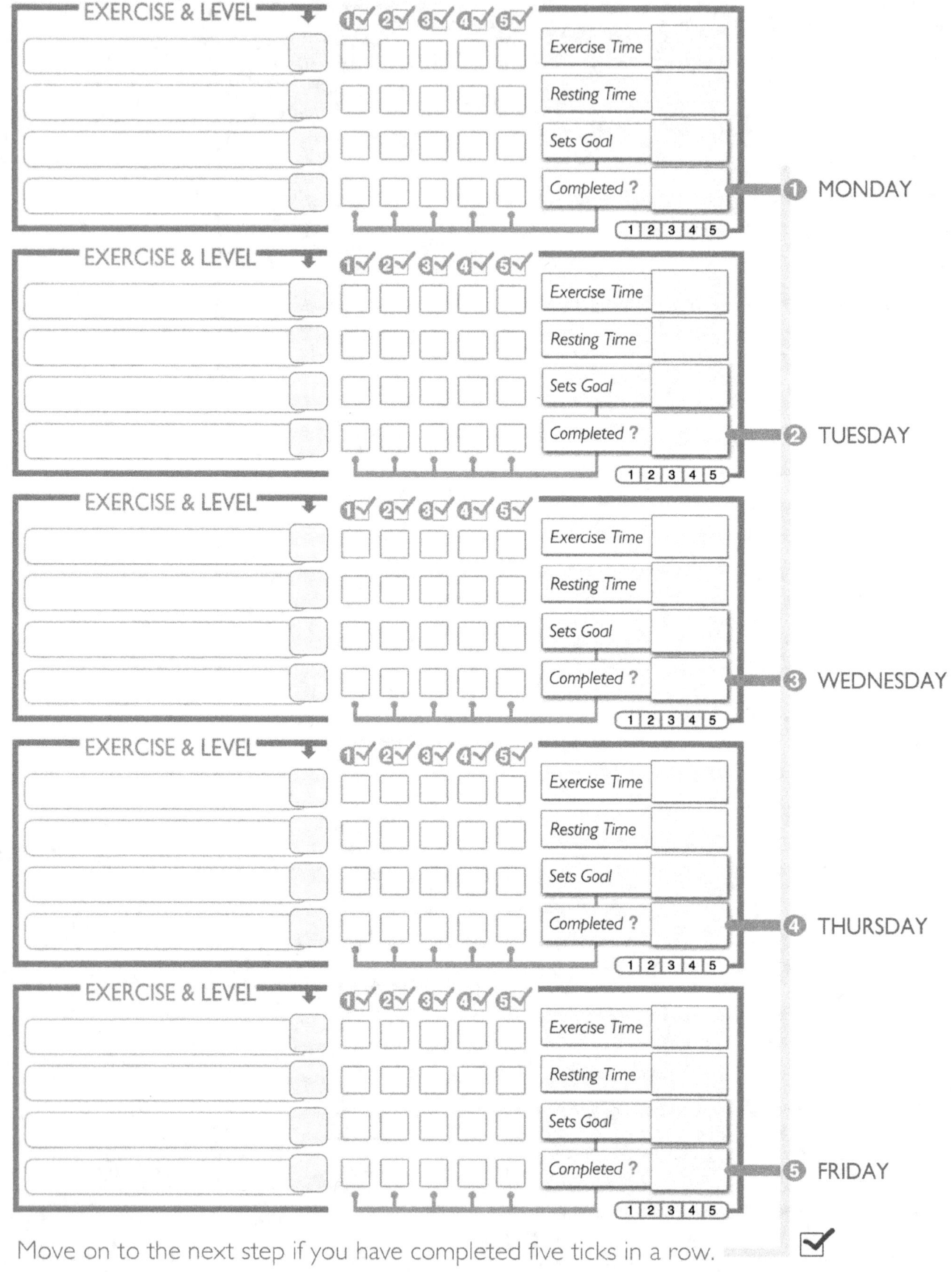

EXERCISE & LEVEL

Exercise Time

Resting Time

Sets Goal

Completed ?

1 2 3 4 5

① MONDAY

EXERCISE & LEVEL

Exercise Time

Resting Time

Sets Goal

Completed ?

1 2 3 4 5

② TUESDAY

EXERCISE & LEVEL

Exercise Time

Resting Time

Sets Goal

Completed ?

1 2 3 4 5

③ WEDNESDAY

EXERCISE & LEVEL

Exercise Time

Resting Time

Sets Goal

Completed ?

1 2 3 4 5

④ THURSDAY

EXERCISE & LEVEL

Exercise Time

Resting Time

Sets Goal

Completed ?

1 2 3 4 5

⑤ FRIDAY

Move on to the next step if you have completed five ticks in a row.

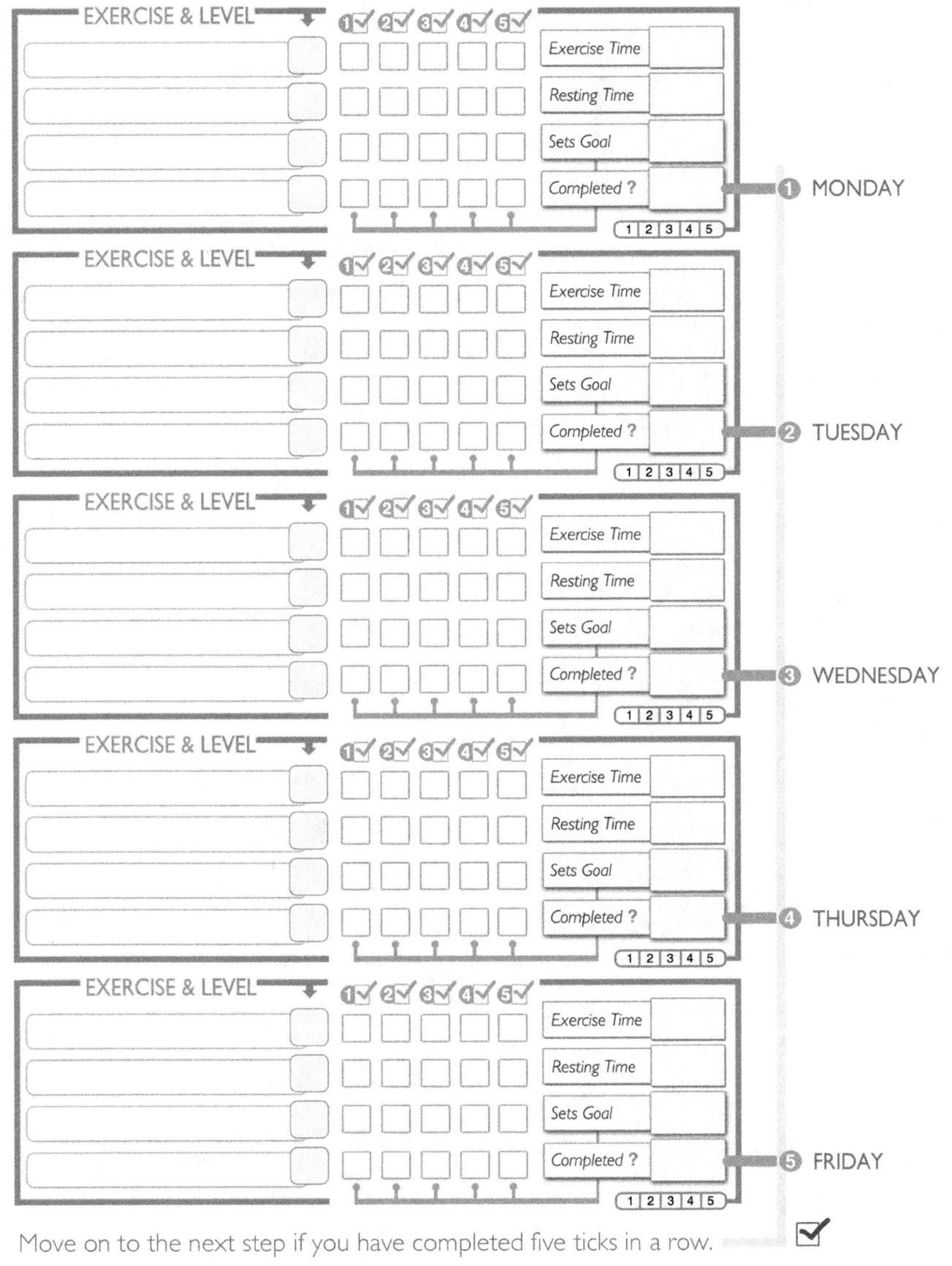

EXERCISE & LEVEL	1✓ 2✓ 3✓ 4✓ 5✓			
		Exercise Time		
		Resting Time		
		Sets Goal		
		Completed ?		❶ MONDAY

1 2 3 4 5

EXERCISE & LEVEL	1✓ 2✓ 3✓ 4✓ 5✓			
		Exercise Time		
		Resting Time		
		Sets Goal		
		Completed ?		❷ TUESDAY

1 2 3 4 5

EXERCISE & LEVEL	1✓ 2✓ 3✓ 4✓ 5✓			
		Exercise Time		
		Resting Time		
		Sets Goal		
		Completed ?		❸ WEDNESDAY

1 2 3 4 5

EXERCISE & LEVEL	1✓ 2✓ 3✓ 4✓ 5✓			
		Exercise Time		
		Resting Time		
		Sets Goal		
		Completed ?		❹ THURSDAY

1 2 3 4 5

EXERCISE & LEVEL	1✓ 2✓ 3✓ 4✓ 5✓			
		Exercise Time		
		Resting Time		
		Sets Goal		
		Completed ?		❺ FRIDAY

1 2 3 4 5

Move on to the next step if you have completed five ticks in a row. ☑

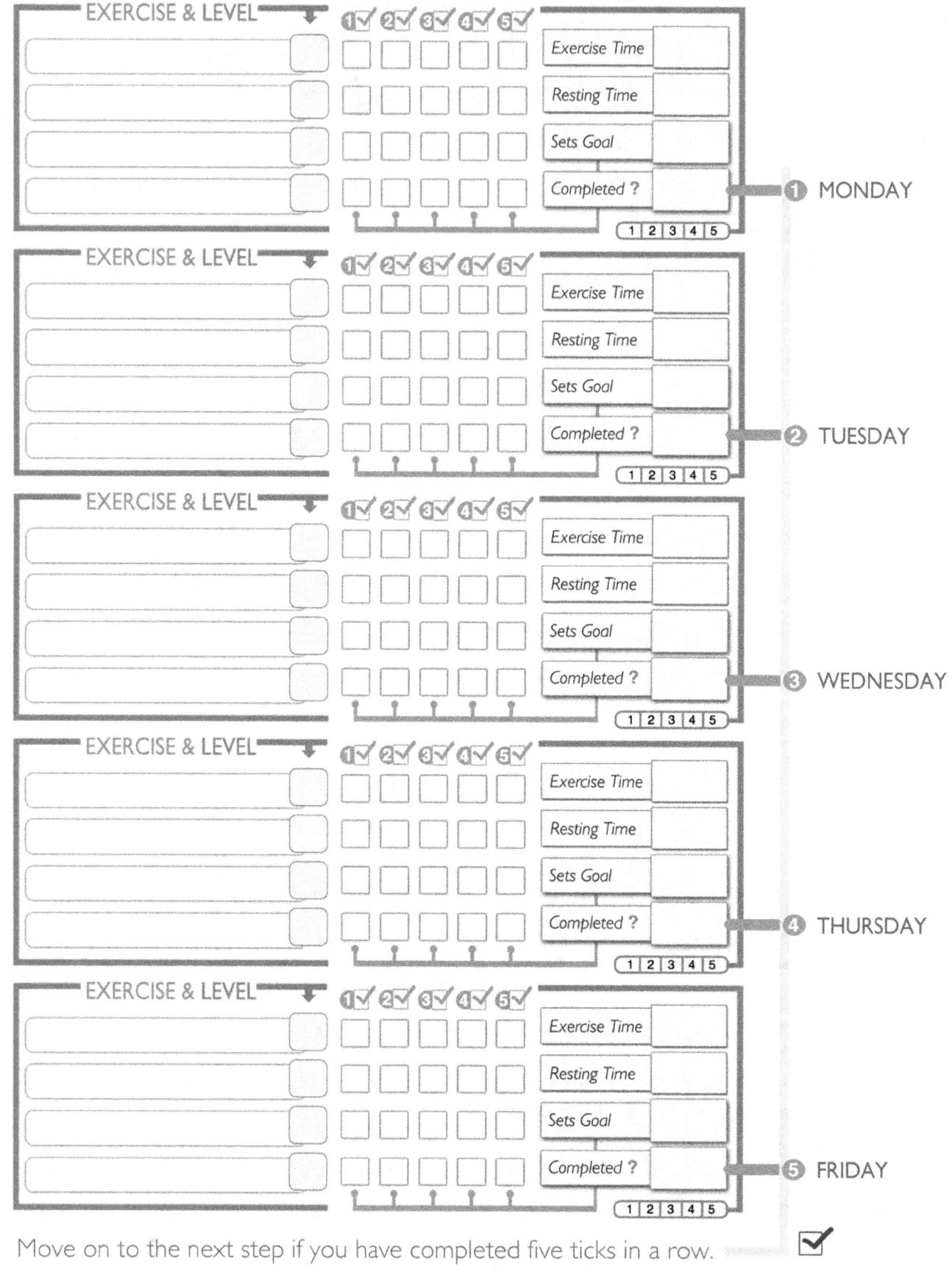

EXERCISE & LEVEL

1☑ 2☑ 3☑ 4☑ 5☑

Exercise Time

Resting Time

Sets Goal

Completed ?

1 2 3 4 5

① MONDAY

EXERCISE & LEVEL

1☑ 2☑ 3☑ 4☑ 5☑

Exercise Time

Resting Time

Sets Goal

Completed ?

1 2 3 4 5

② TUESDAY

EXERCISE & LEVEL

1☑ 2☑ 3☑ 4☑ 5☑

Exercise Time

Resting Time

Sets Goal

Completed ?

1 2 3 4 5

③ WEDNESDAY

EXERCISE & LEVEL

1☑ 2☑ 3☑ 4☑ 5☑

Exercise Time

Resting Time

Sets Goal

Completed ?

1 2 3 4 5

④ THURSDAY

EXERCISE & LEVEL

1☑ 2☑ 3☑ 4☑ 5☑

Exercise Time

Resting Time

Sets Goal

Completed ?

1 2 3 4 5

⑤ FRIDAY

Move on to the next step if you have completed five ticks in a row. ☑

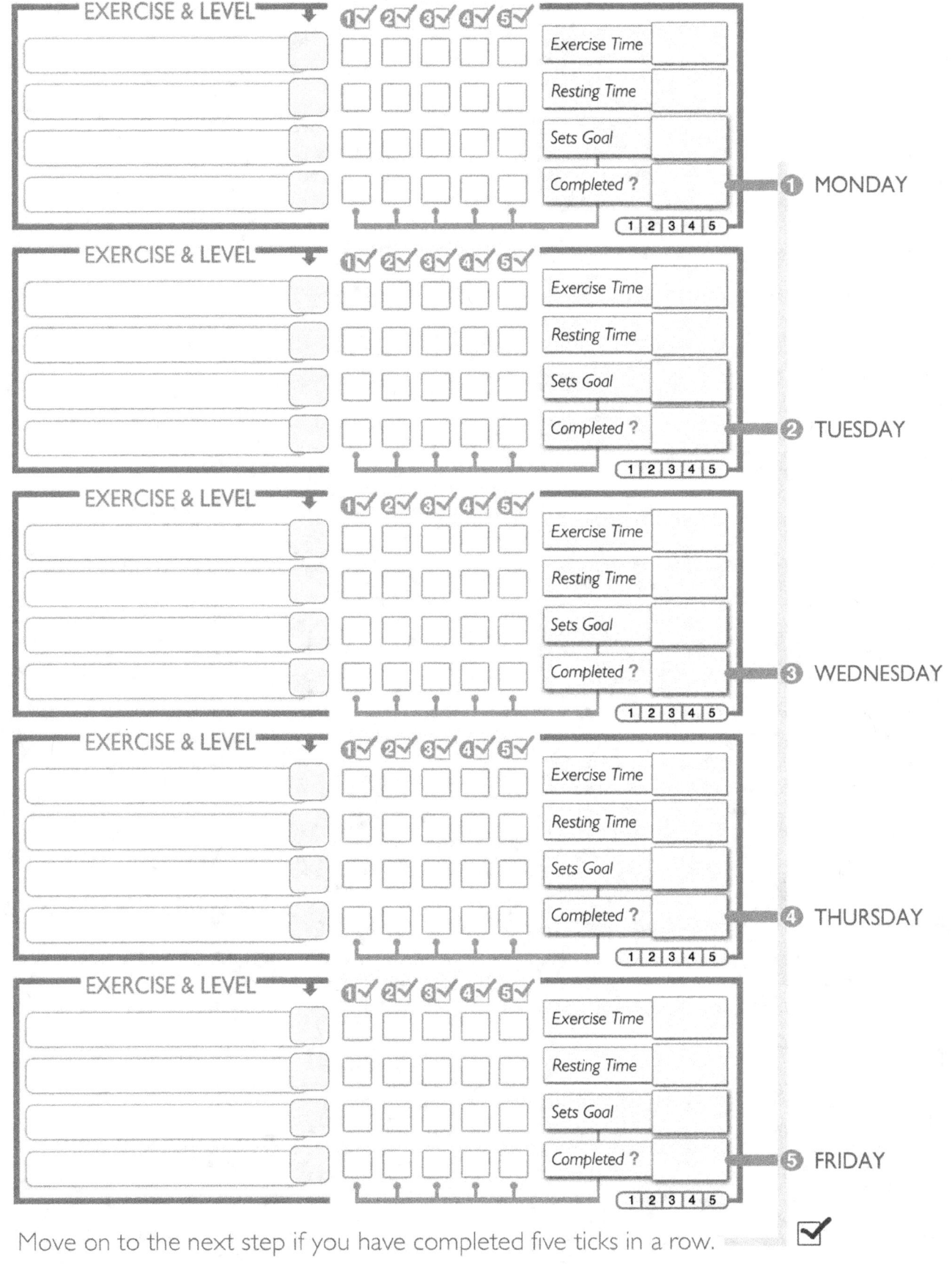

Move on to the next step if you have completed five ticks in a row.

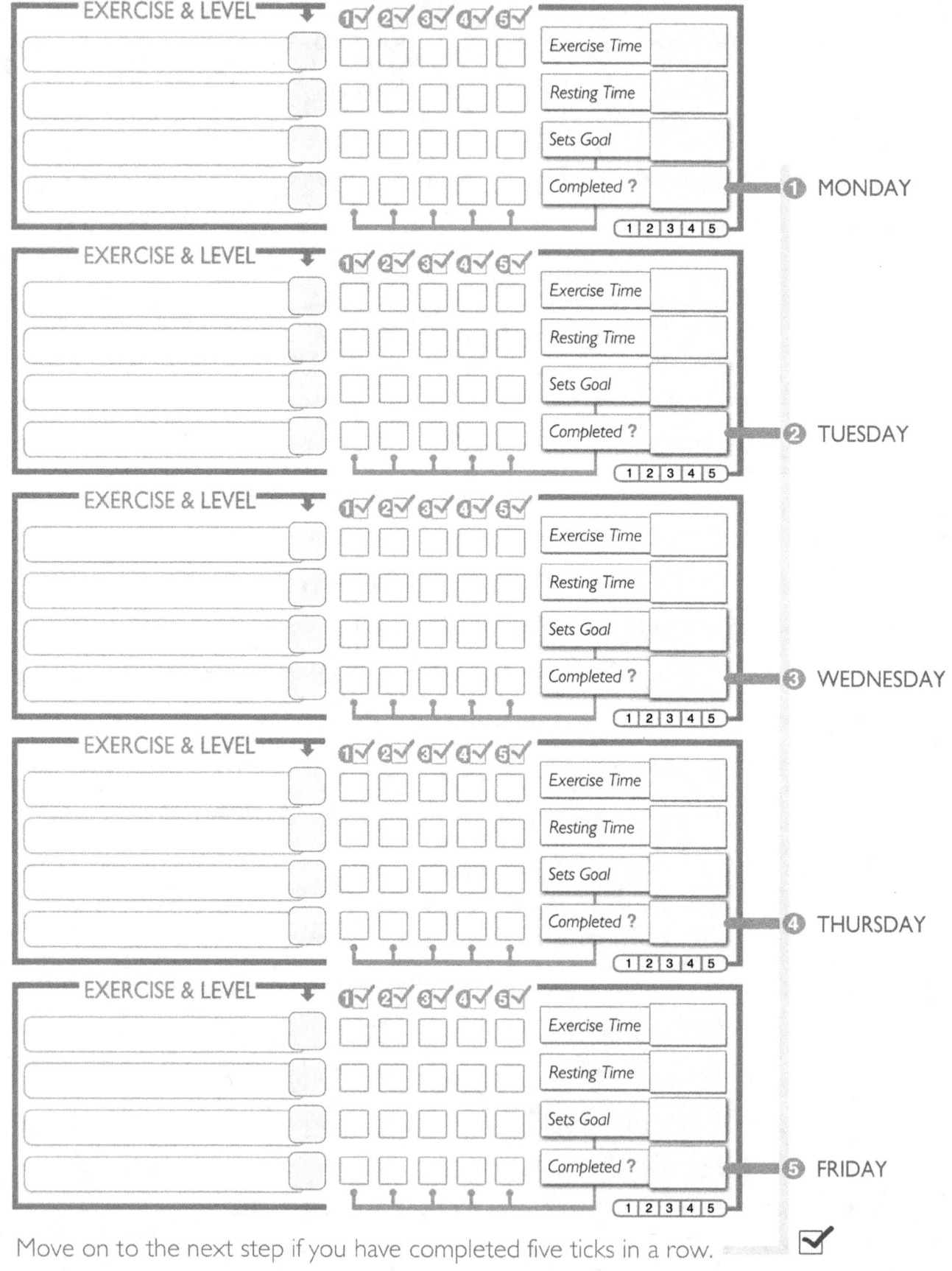

EXERCISE & LEVEL ❶✓ ❷✓ ❸✓ ❹✓ ❺✓

Exercise Time
Resting Time
Sets Goal
Completed ?

❶ MONDAY

1 2 3 4 5

EXERCISE & LEVEL ❶✓ ❷✓ ❸✓ ❹✓ ❺✓

Exercise Time
Resting Time
Sets Goal
Completed ?

❷ TUESDAY

1 2 3 4 5

EXERCISE & LEVEL ❶✓ ❷✓ ❸✓ ❹✓ ❺✓

Exercise Time
Resting Time
Sets Goal
Completed ?

❸ WEDNESDAY

1 2 3 4 5

EXERCISE & LEVEL ❶✓ ❷✓ ❸✓ ❹✓ ❺✓

Exercise Time
Resting Time
Sets Goal
Completed ?

❹ THURSDAY

1 2 3 4 5

EXERCISE & LEVEL ❶✓ ❷✓ ❸✓ ❹✓ ❺✓

Exercise Time
Resting Time
Sets Goal
Completed ?

❺ FRIDAY

1 2 3 4 5

Move on to the next step if you have completed five ticks in a row. ☑

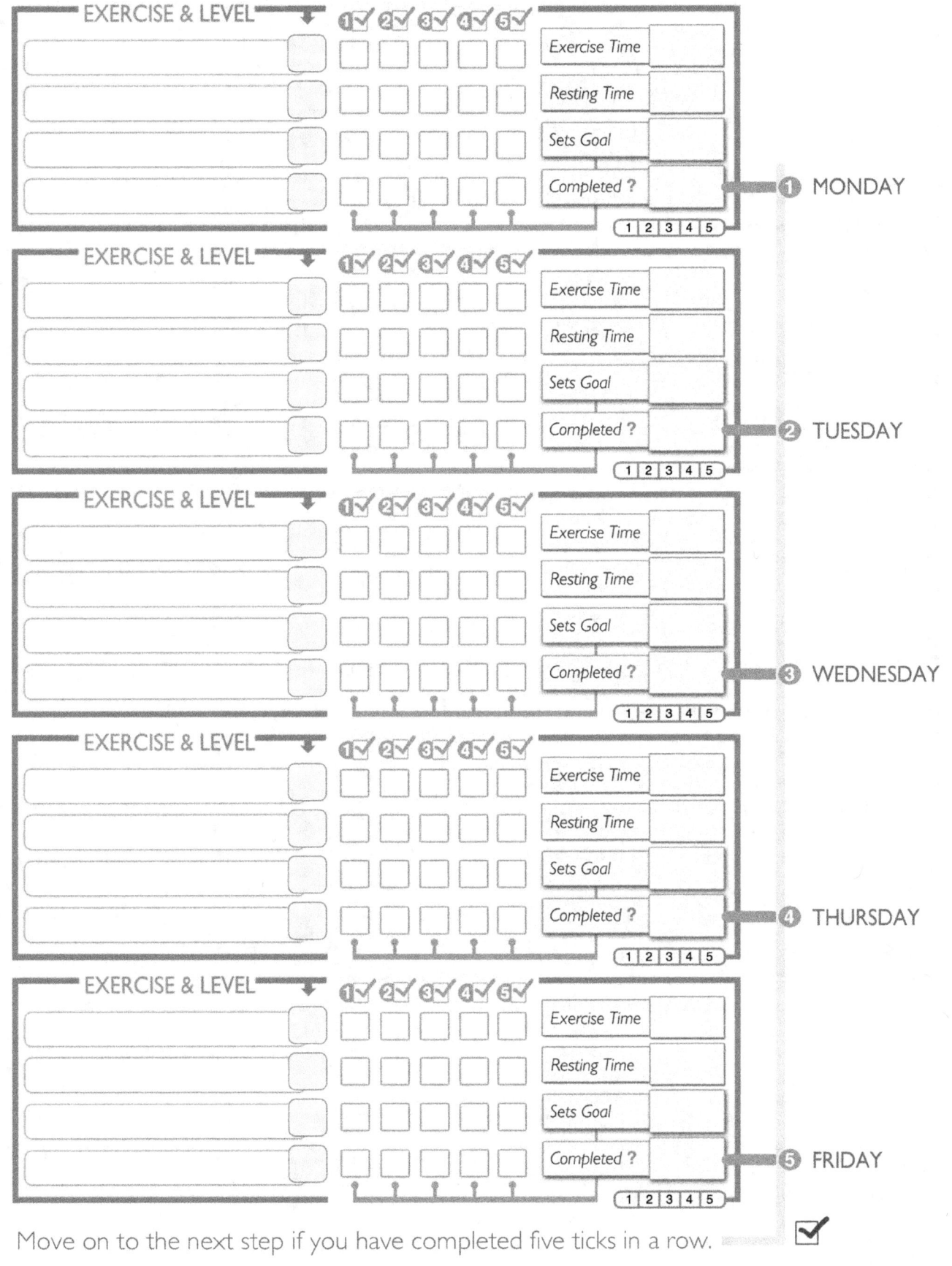

EXERCISE & LEVEL

| 1 ✓ | 2 ✓ | 3 ✓ | 4 ✓ | 5 ✓ |

Exercise Time
Resting Time
Sets Goal
Completed ?

1 2 3 4 5

❶ MONDAY

EXERCISE & LEVEL

| 1 ✓ | 2 ✓ | 3 ✓ | 4 ✓ | 5 ✓ |

Exercise Time
Resting Time
Sets Goal
Completed ?

1 2 3 4 5

❷ TUESDAY

EXERCISE & LEVEL

| 1 ✓ | 2 ✓ | 3 ✓ | 4 ✓ | 5 ✓ |

Exercise Time
Resting Time
Sets Goal
Completed ?

1 2 3 4 5

❸ WEDNESDAY

EXERCISE & LEVEL

| 1 ✓ | 2 ✓ | 3 ✓ | 4 ✓ | 5 ✓ |

Exercise Time
Resting Time
Sets Goal
Completed ?

1 2 3 4 5

❹ THURSDAY

EXERCISE & LEVEL

| 1 ✓ | 2 ✓ | 3 ✓ | 4 ✓ | 5 ✓ |

Exercise Time
Resting Time
Sets Goal
Completed ?

1 2 3 4 5

❺ FRIDAY

Move on to the next step if you have completed five ticks in a row. ☑

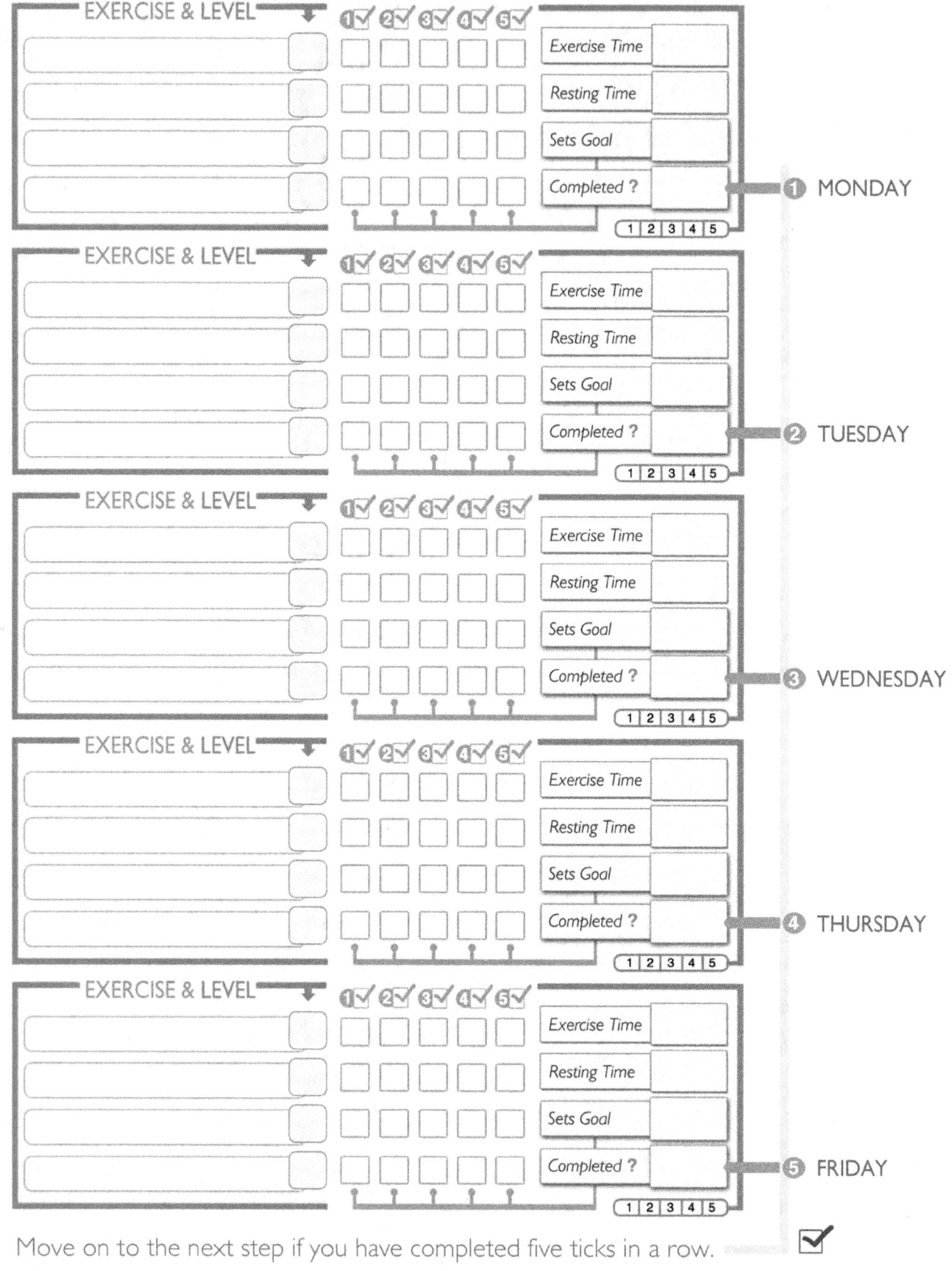

Move on to the next step if you have completed five ticks in a row.

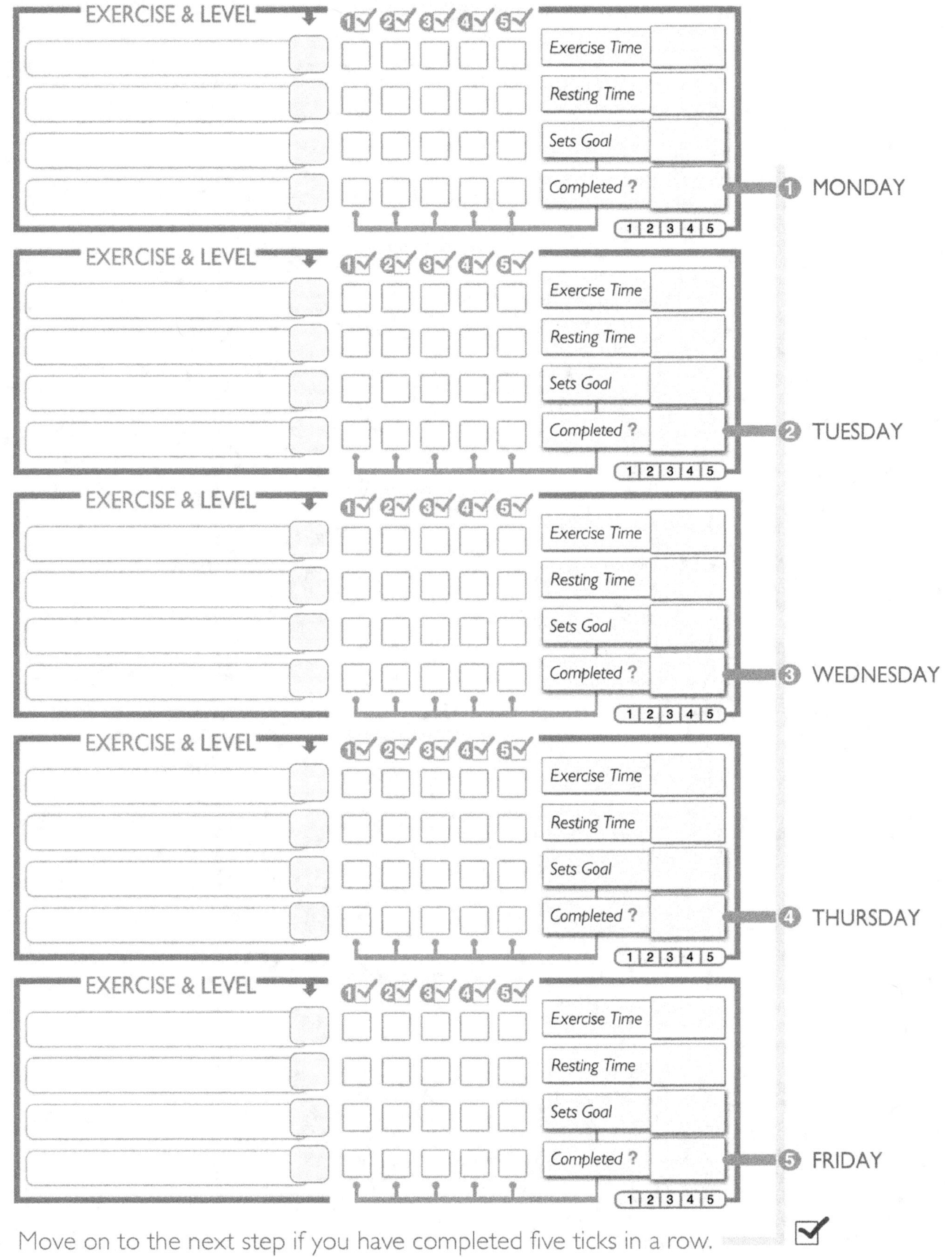

EXERCISE & LEVEL

| | 1 ✓ | 2 ✓ | 3 ✓ | 4 ✓ | 5 ✓ |

Exercise Time
Resting Time
Sets Goal
Completed ?

1 MONDAY

1 2 3 4 5

EXERCISE & LEVEL

| | 1 ✓ | 2 ✓ | 3 ✓ | 4 ✓ | 5 ✓ |

Exercise Time
Resting Time
Sets Goal
Completed ?

2 TUESDAY

1 2 3 4 5

EXERCISE & LEVEL

| | 1 ✓ | 2 ✓ | 3 ✓ | 4 ✓ | 5 ✓ |

Exercise Time
Resting Time
Sets Goal
Completed ?

3 WEDNESDAY

1 2 3 4 5

EXERCISE & LEVEL

| | 1 ✓ | 2 ✓ | 3 ✓ | 4 ✓ | 5 ✓ |

Exercise Time
Resting Time
Sets Goal
Completed ?

4 THURSDAY

1 2 3 4 5

EXERCISE & LEVEL

| | 1 ✓ | 2 ✓ | 3 ✓ | 4 ✓ | 5 ✓ |

Exercise Time
Resting Time
Sets Goal
Completed ?

5 FRIDAY

1 2 3 4 5

Move on to the next step if you have completed five ticks in a row. ☑

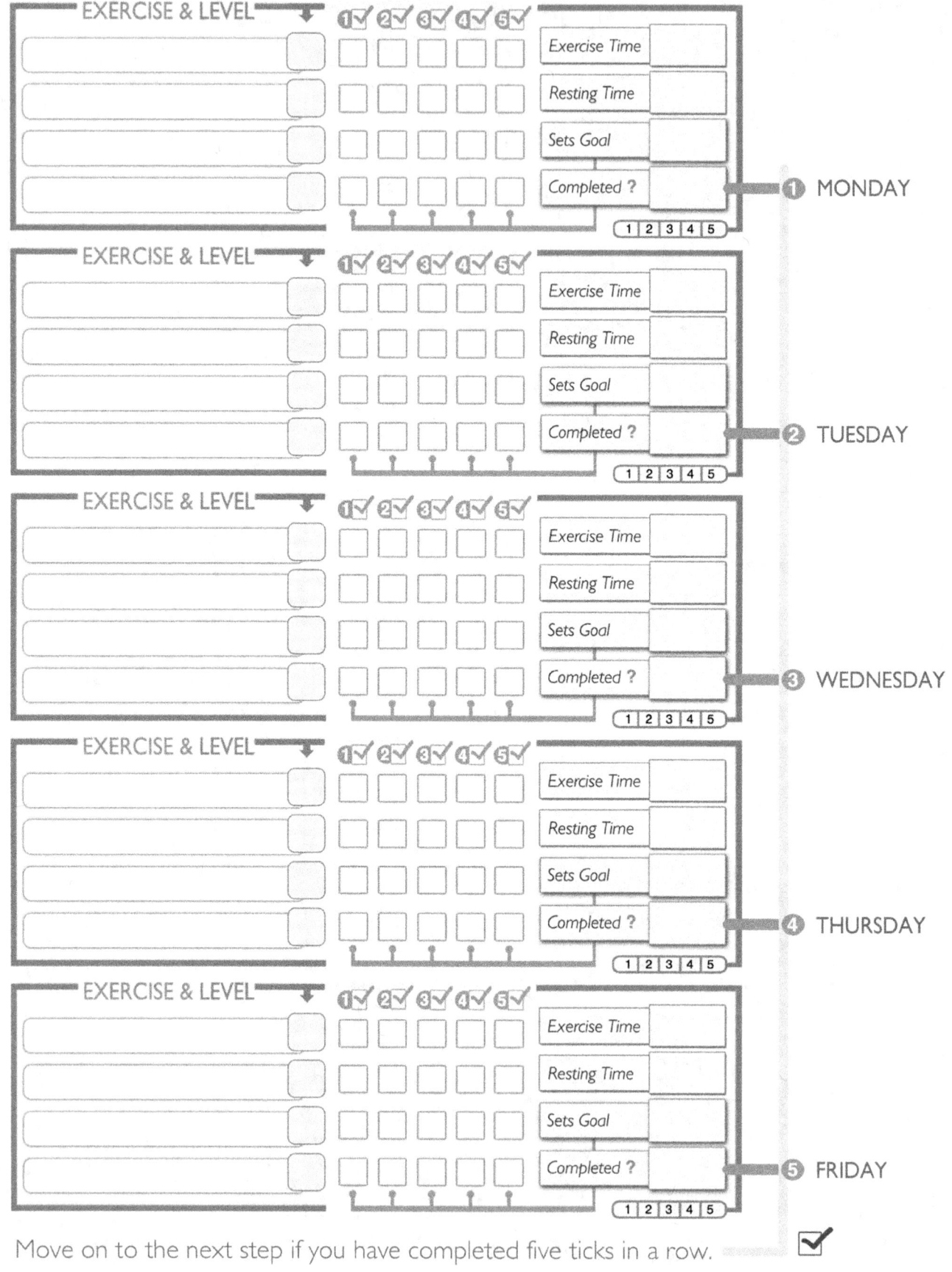

EXERCISE & LEVEL ☑1 ☑2 ☑3 ☑4 ☑5

Exercise Time
Resting Time
Sets Goal
Completed ?

1 2 3 4 5

1 MONDAY

Exercise Time
Resting Time
Sets Goal
Completed ?

1 2 3 4 5

2 TUESDAY

Exercise Time
Resting Time
Sets Goal
Completed ?

1 2 3 4 5

3 WEDNESDAY

Exercise Time
Resting Time
Sets Goal
Completed ?

1 2 3 4 5

4 THURSDAY

Exercise Time
Resting Time
Sets Goal
Completed ?

1 2 3 4 5

5 FRIDAY

Move on to the next step if you have completed five ticks in a row. ☑

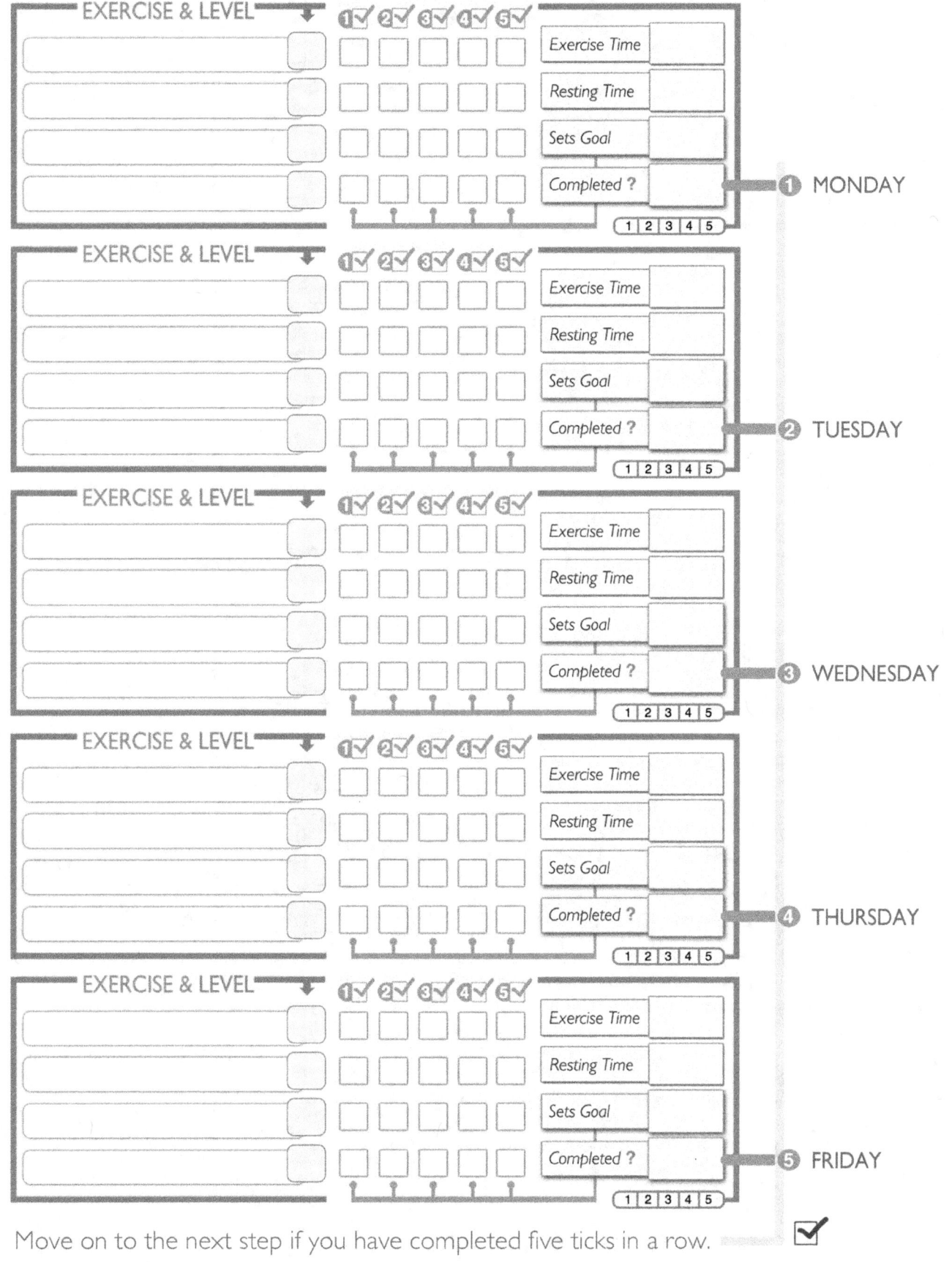

EXERCISE & LEVEL

1✓ 2✓ 3✓ 4✓ 5✓

Exercise Time

Resting Time

Sets Goal

Completed ?

1 | 2 | 3 | 4 | 5

1 MONDAY

EXERCISE & LEVEL

1✓ 2✓ 3✓ 4✓ 5✓

Exercise Time

Resting Time

Sets Goal

Completed ?

1 | 2 | 3 | 4 | 5

2 TUESDAY

EXERCISE & LEVEL

1✓ 2✓ 3✓ 4✓ 5✓

Exercise Time

Resting Time

Sets Goal

Completed ?

1 | 2 | 3 | 4 | 5

3 WEDNESDAY

EXERCISE & LEVEL

1✓ 2✓ 3✓ 4✓ 5✓

Exercise Time

Resting Time

Sets Goal

Completed ?

1 | 2 | 3 | 4 | 5

4 THURSDAY

EXERCISE & LEVEL

1✓ 2✓ 3✓ 4✓ 5✓

Exercise Time

Resting Time

Sets Goal

Completed ?

1 | 2 | 3 | 4 | 5

5 FRIDAY

Move on to the next step if you have completed five ticks in a row. ☑

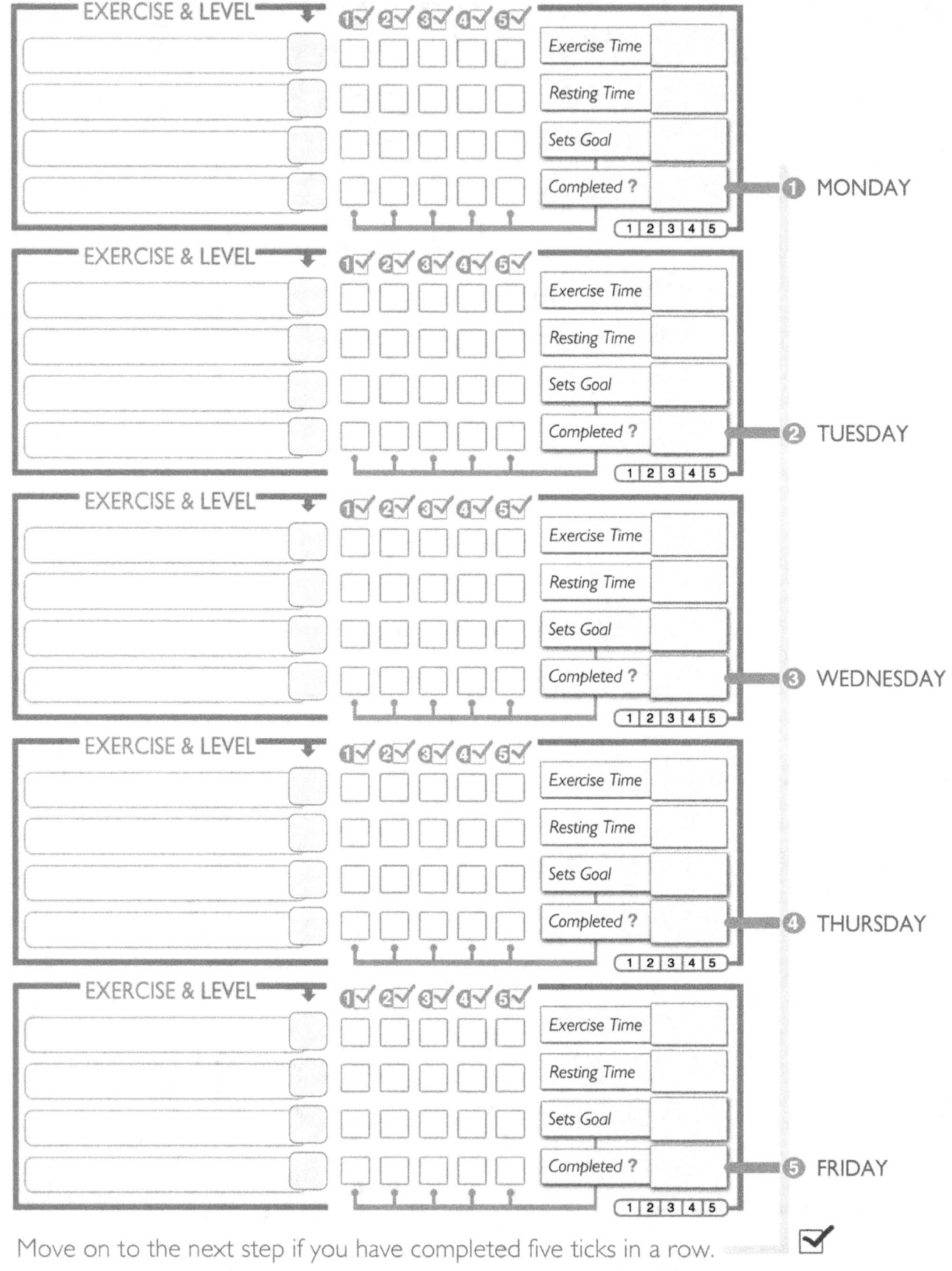

EXERCISE & LEVEL — 1✓ 2✓ 3✓ 4✓ 5✓

Exercise Time
Resting Time
Sets Goal
Completed ?

1 MONDAY
1 2 3 4 5

EXERCISE & LEVEL — 1✓ 2✓ 3✓ 4✓ 5✓

Exercise Time
Resting Time
Sets Goal
Completed ?

2 TUESDAY
1 2 3 4 5

EXERCISE & LEVEL — 1✓ 2✓ 3✓ 4✓ 5✓

Exercise Time
Resting Time
Sets Goal
Completed ?

3 WEDNESDAY
1 2 3 4 5

EXERCISE & LEVEL — 1✓ 2✓ 3✓ 4✓ 5✓

Exercise Time
Resting Time
Sets Goal
Completed ?

4 THURSDAY
1 2 3 4 5

EXERCISE & LEVEL — 1✓ 2✓ 3✓ 4✓ 5✓

Exercise Time
Resting Time
Sets Goal
Completed ?

5 FRIDAY
1 2 3 4 5

Move on to the next step if you have completed five ticks in a row. ☑

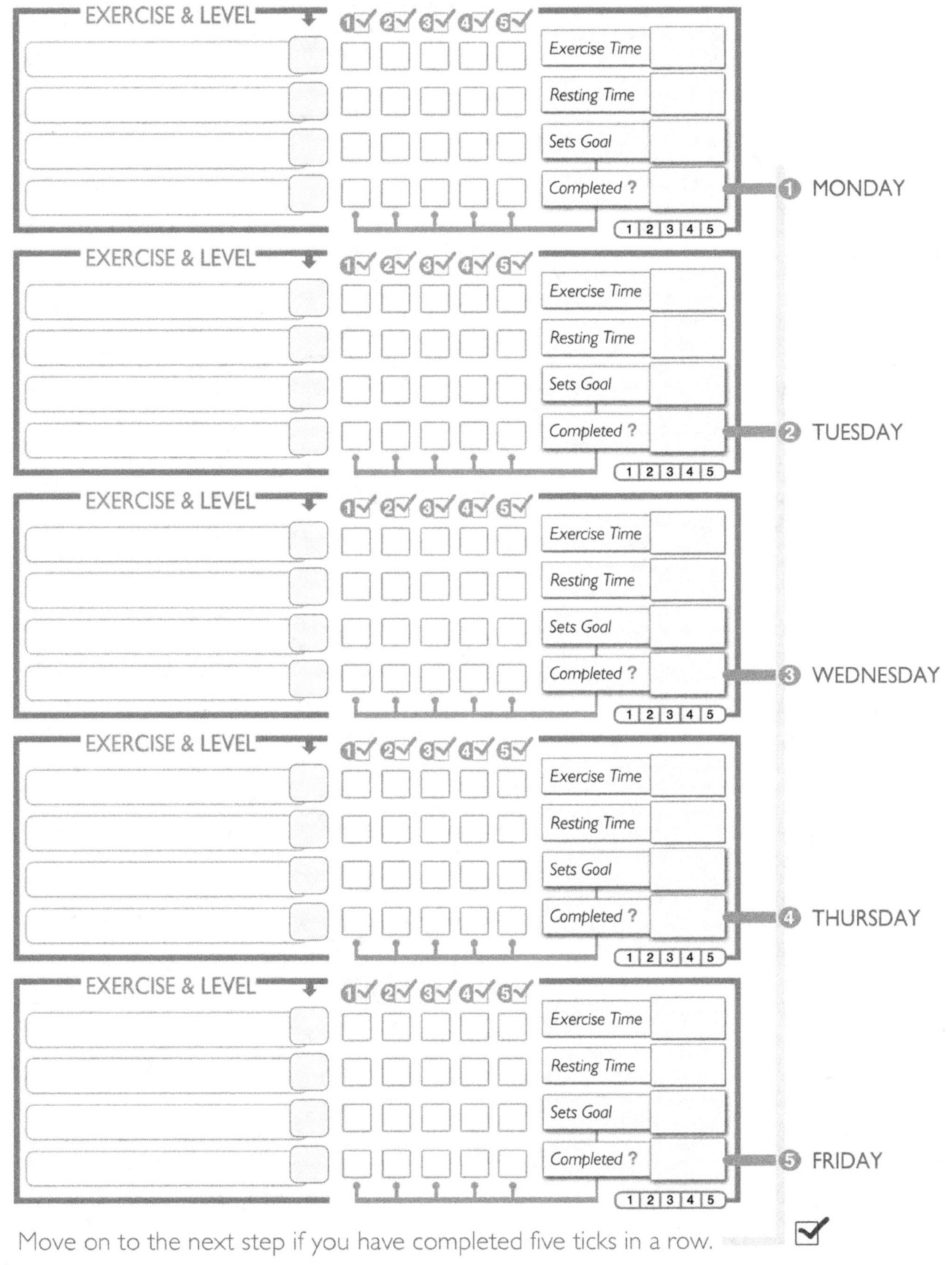

EXERCISE & LEVEL ① ✓ ② ✓ ③ ✓ ④ ✓ ⑤ ✓

Exercise Time
Resting Time
Sets Goal
Completed ?

❶ MONDAY

1 2 3 4 5

EXERCISE & LEVEL ① ✓ ② ✓ ③ ✓ ④ ✓ ⑤ ✓

Exercise Time
Resting Time
Sets Goal
Completed ?

❷ TUESDAY

1 2 3 4 5

EXERCISE & LEVEL ① ✓ ② ✓ ③ ✓ ④ ✓ ⑤ ✓

Exercise Time
Resting Time
Sets Goal
Completed ?

❸ WEDNESDAY

1 2 3 4 5

EXERCISE & LEVEL ① ✓ ② ✓ ③ ✓ ④ ✓ ⑤ ✓

Exercise Time
Resting Time
Sets Goal
Completed ?

❹ THURSDAY

1 2 3 4 5

EXERCISE & LEVEL ① ✓ ② ✓ ③ ✓ ④ ✓ ⑤ ✓

Exercise Time
Resting Time
Sets Goal
Completed ?

❺ FRIDAY

1 2 3 4 5

Move on to the next step if you have completed five ticks in a row. ✓

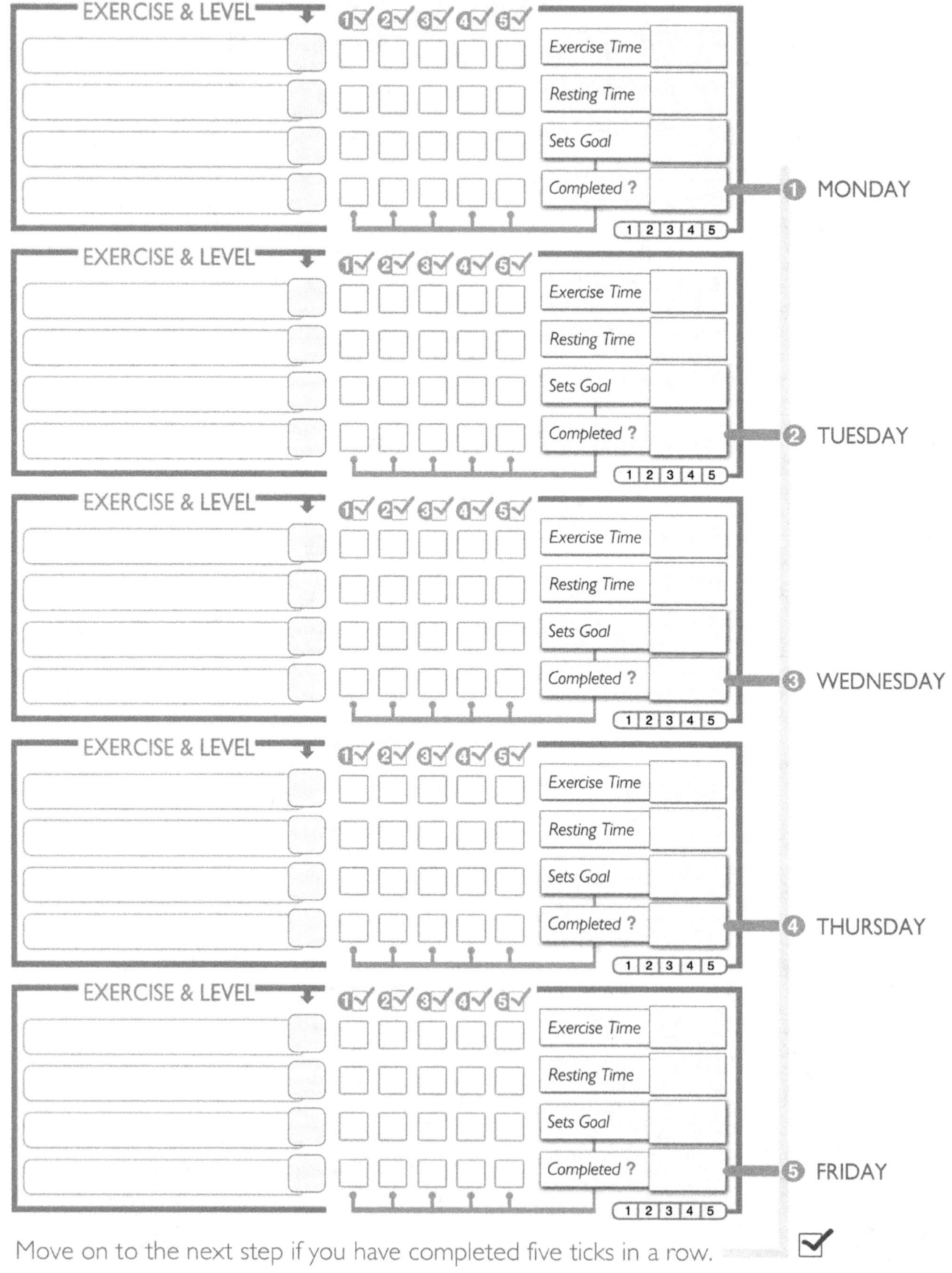

Move on to the next step if you have completed five ticks in a row.

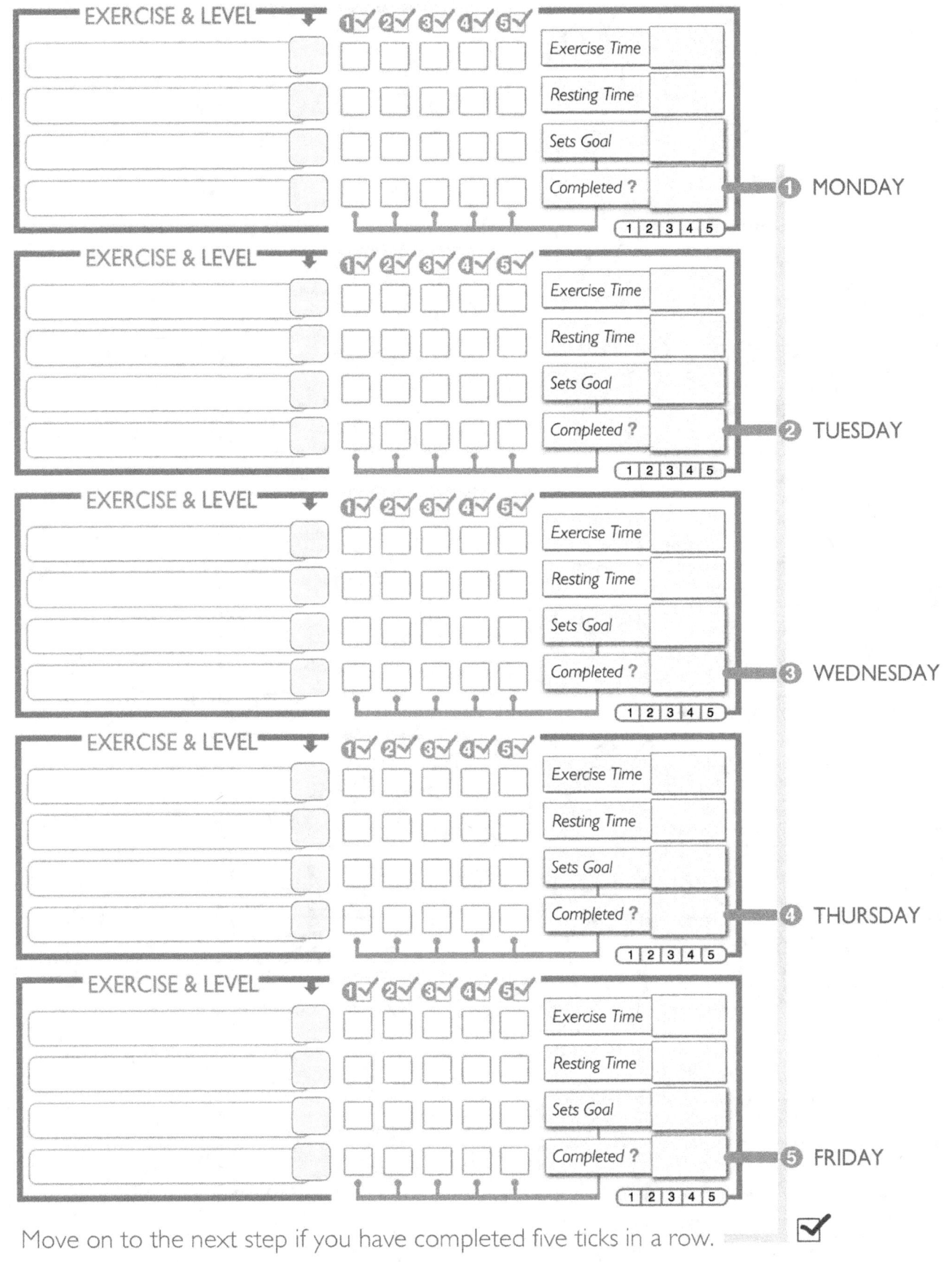

Move on to the next step if you have completed five ticks in a row.

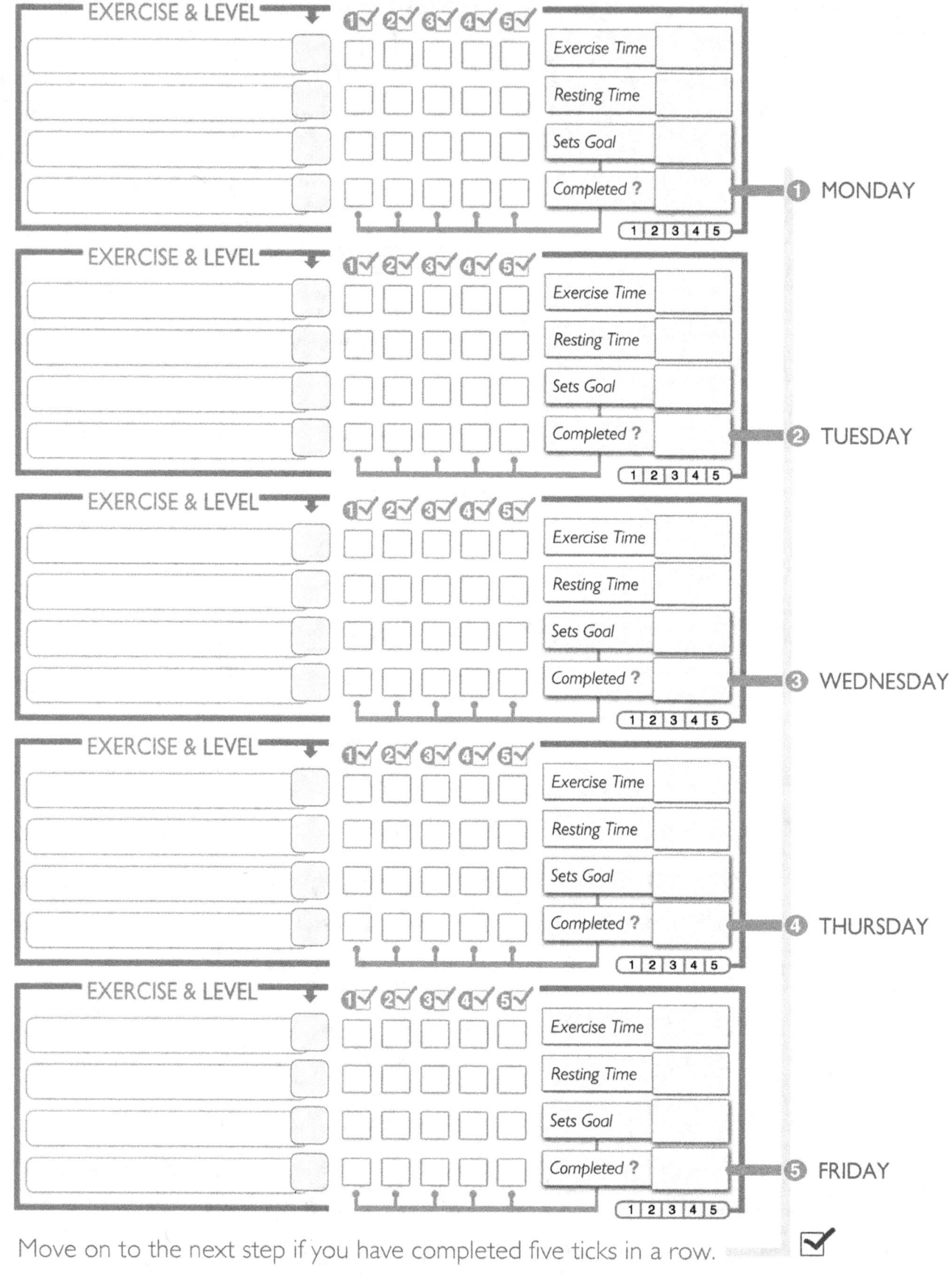

EXERCISE & LEVEL ▼ 1✓ 2✓ 3✓ 4✓ 5✓

Exercise Time
Resting Time
Sets Goal
Completed ?

❶ MONDAY

1 2 3 4 5

EXERCISE & LEVEL ▼ 1✓ 2✓ 3✓ 4✓ 5✓

Exercise Time
Resting Time
Sets Goal
Completed ?

❷ TUESDAY

1 2 3 4 5

EXERCISE & LEVEL ▼ 1✓ 2✓ 3✓ 4✓ 5✓

Exercise Time
Resting Time
Sets Goal
Completed ?

❸ WEDNESDAY

1 2 3 4 5

EXERCISE & LEVEL ▼ 1✓ 2✓ 3✓ 4✓ 5✓

Exercise Time
Resting Time
Sets Goal
Completed ?

❹ THURSDAY

1 2 3 4 5

EXERCISE & LEVEL ▼ 1✓ 2✓ 3✓ 4✓ 5✓

Exercise Time
Resting Time
Sets Goal
Completed ?

❺ FRIDAY

1 2 3 4 5

Move on to the next step if you have completed five ticks in a row. ☑

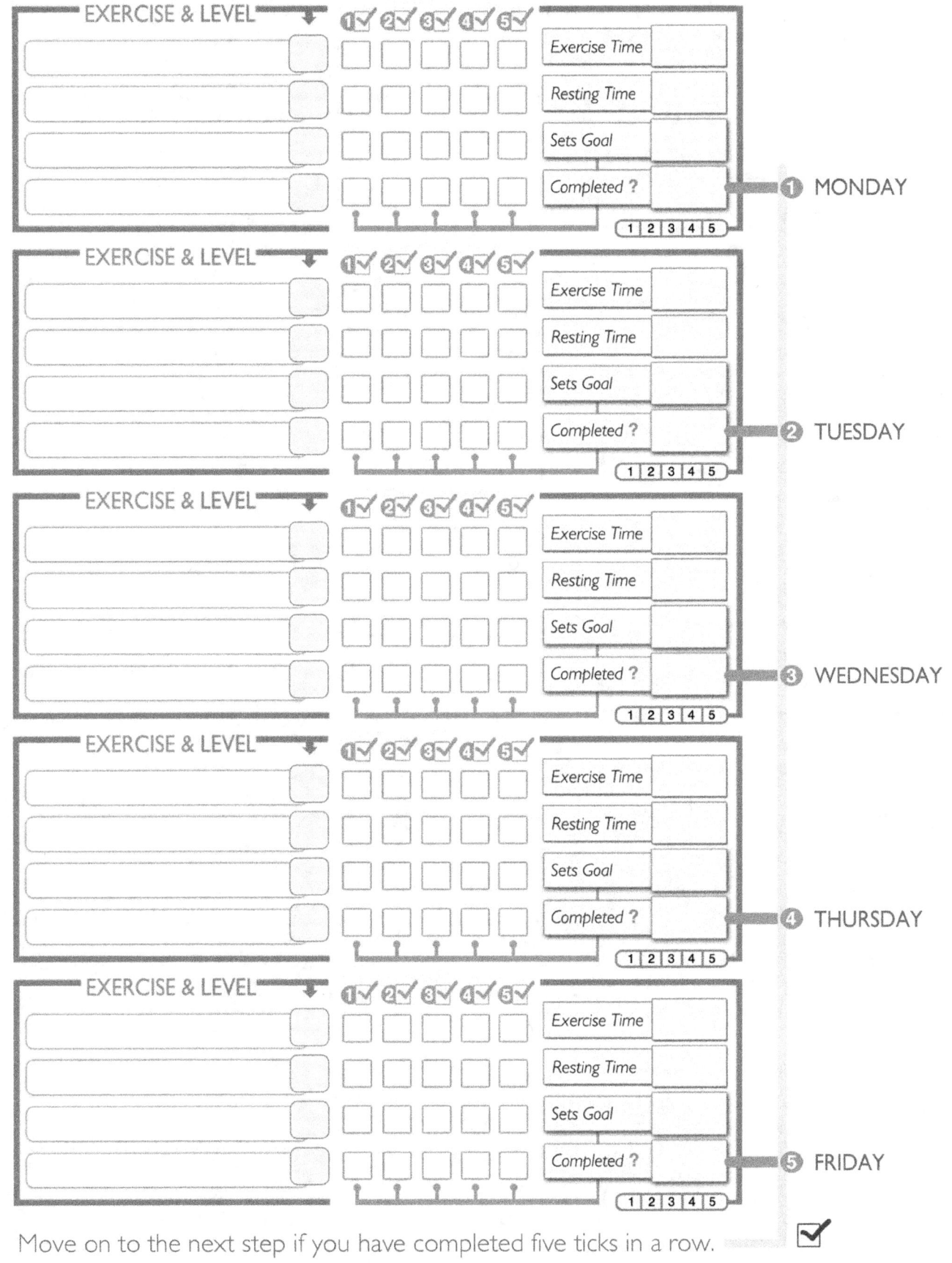

Move on to the next step if you have completed five ticks in a row.

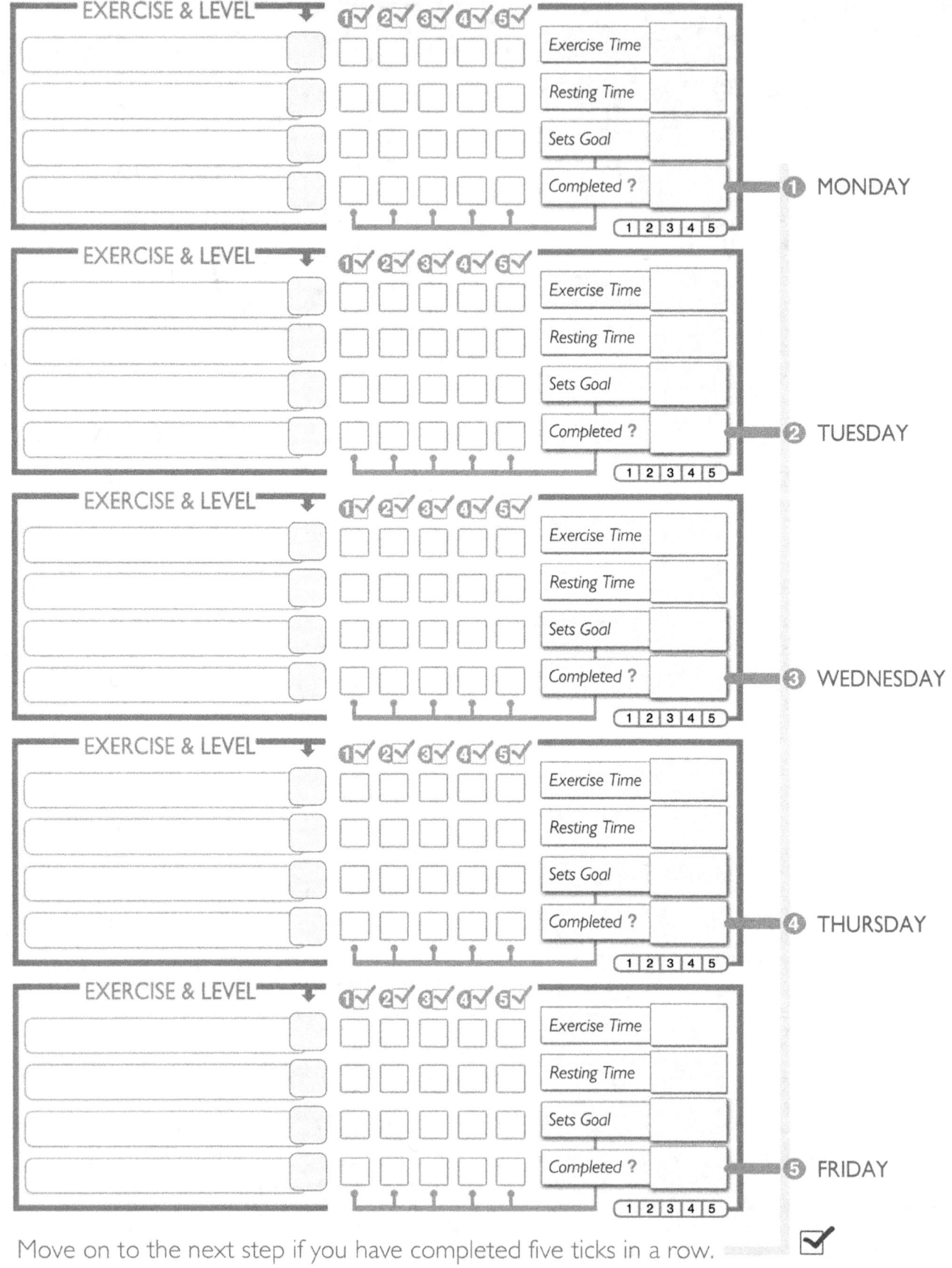

Move on to the next step if you have completed five ticks in a row. ☑

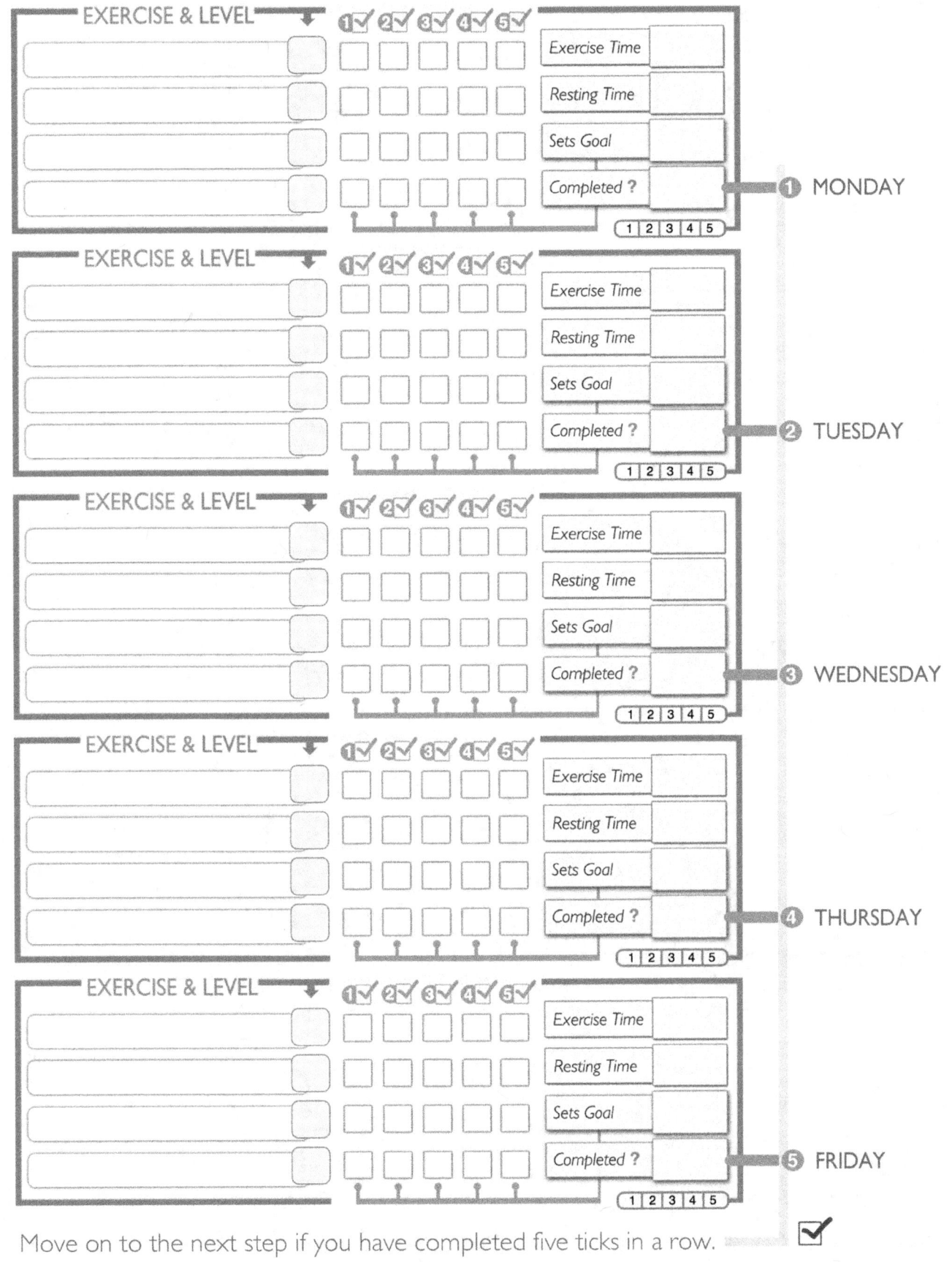

EXERCISE & LEVEL

	1☑	2☑	3☑	4☑	5☑

Exercise Time

Resting Time

Sets Goal

Completed ?

1 2 3 4 5

1 MONDAY

2 TUESDAY

3 WEDNESDAY

4 THURSDAY

5 FRIDAY

Move on to the next step if you have completed five ticks in a row. ☑

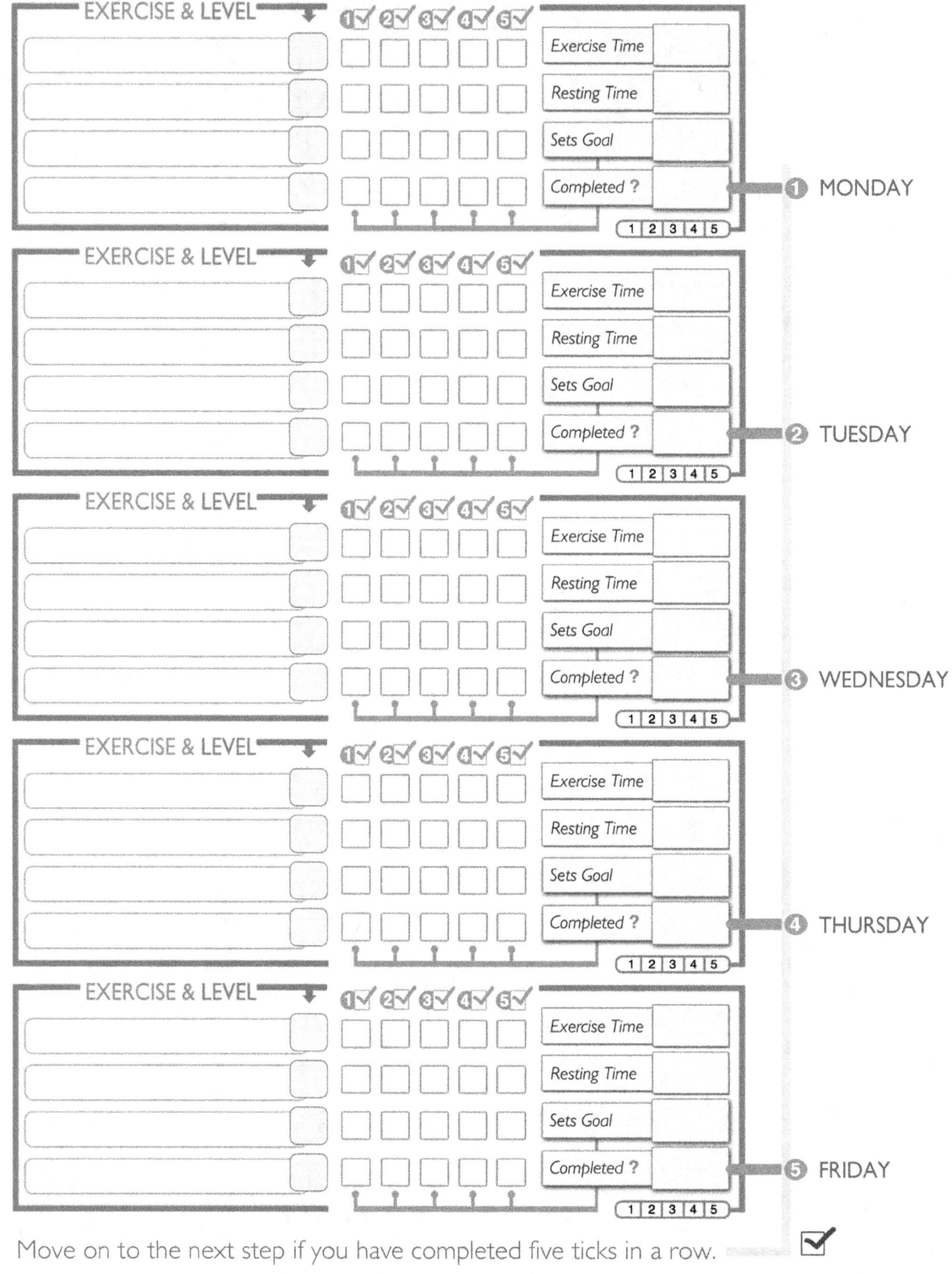

EXERCISE & LEVEL ① ② ③ ④ ⑤ Exercise Time Resting Time Sets Goal Completed ? **1** MONDAY 1 2 3 4 5

EXERCISE & LEVEL ① ② ③ ④ ⑤ Exercise Time Resting Time Sets Goal Completed ? **2** TUESDAY 1 2 3 4 5

EXERCISE & LEVEL ① ② ③ ④ ⑤ Exercise Time Resting Time Sets Goal Completed ? **3** WEDNESDAY 1 2 3 4 5

EXERCISE & LEVEL ① ② ③ ④ ⑤ Exercise Time Resting Time Sets Goal Completed ? **4** THURSDAY 1 2 3 4 5

EXERCISE & LEVEL ① ② ③ ④ ⑤ Exercise Time Resting Time Sets Goal Completed ? **5** FRIDAY 1 2 3 4 5

Move on to the next step if you have completed five ticks in a row.

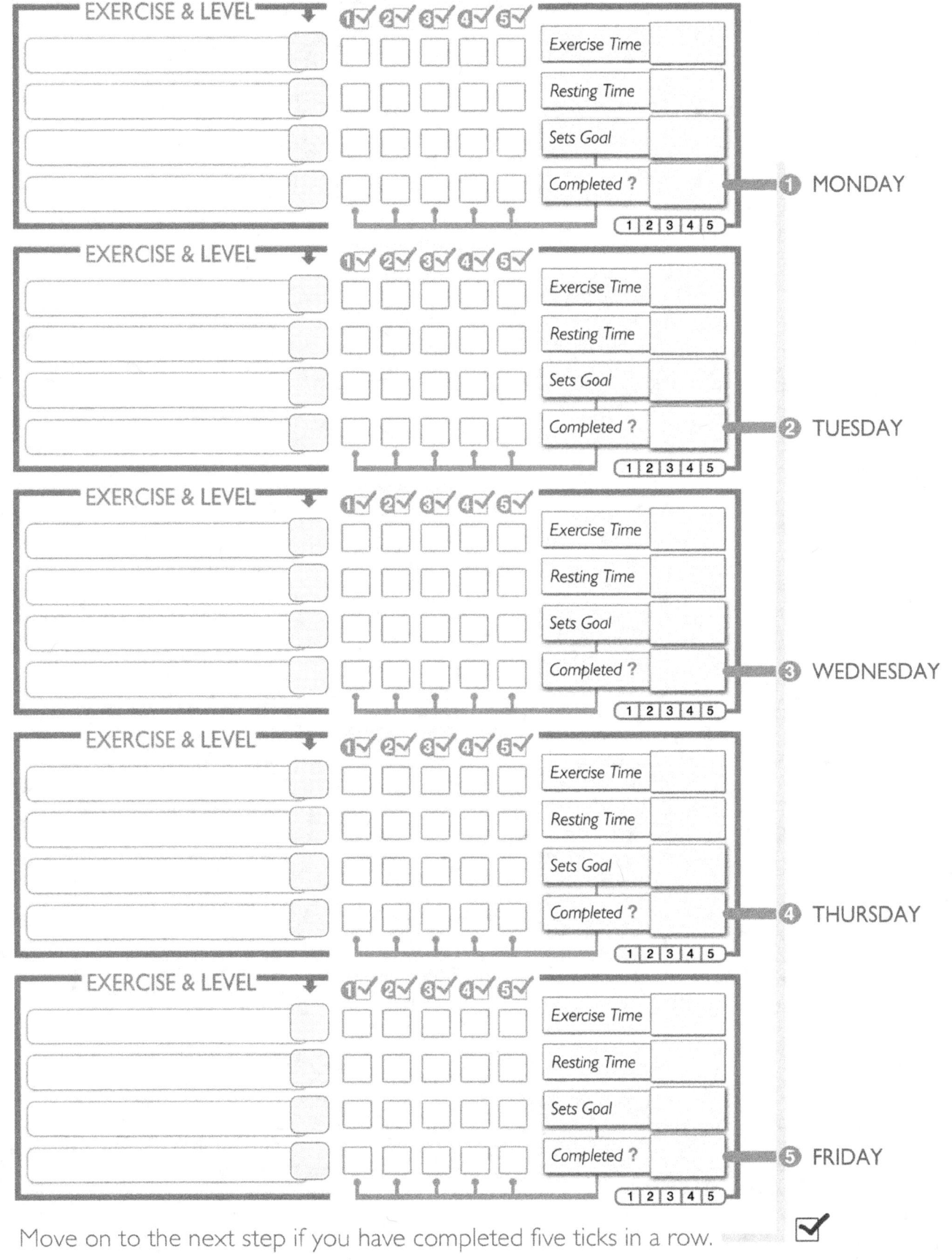

EXERCISE & LEVEL

1 ✓ 2 ✓ 3 ✓ 4 ✓ 5 ✓

Exercise Time
Resting Time
Sets Goal
Completed ?

1 2 3 4 5

❶ MONDAY

EXERCISE & LEVEL

1 ✓ 2 ✓ 3 ✓ 4 ✓ 5 ✓

Exercise Time
Resting Time
Sets Goal
Completed ?

1 2 3 4 5

❷ TUESDAY

EXERCISE & LEVEL

1 ✓ 2 ✓ 3 ✓ 4 ✓ 5 ✓

Exercise Time
Resting Time
Sets Goal
Completed ?

1 2 3 4 5

❸ WEDNESDAY

EXERCISE & LEVEL

1 ✓ 2 ✓ 3 ✓ 4 ✓ 5 ✓

Exercise Time
Resting Time
Sets Goal
Completed ?

1 2 3 4 5

❹ THURSDAY

EXERCISE & LEVEL

1 ✓ 2 ✓ 3 ✓ 4 ✓ 5 ✓

Exercise Time
Resting Time
Sets Goal
Completed ?

1 2 3 4 5

❺ FRIDAY

Move on to the next step if you have completed five ticks in a row. ☑